# HAIR
# Secrets

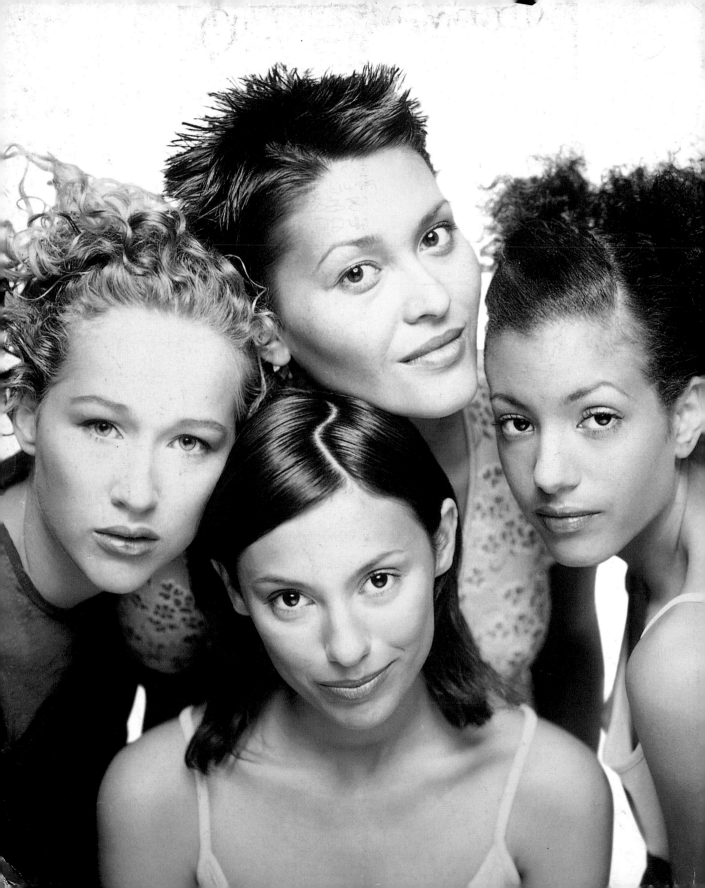

# HAIR
# Secrets

## MAGGIE JONES

FOREWORD BY MARILYN SHERLOCK MIT MAE

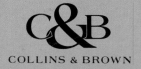

COLLINS & BROWN

First published in Great Britain in 2000
by Collins & Brown Limited
London House
Great Eastern Wharf
Parkgate Road
London SW11 4NQ

Distributed in the United States and Canada by Sterling Publishing Co.
387 Park Avenue South, New York, NY 10016  USA

1 3 5 7 9 8 6 4 2

British Library Cataloguing-in-Publication Data:
A catalogue record for this book is available from the British Library.

ISBN 1 85585 793 6

Designed by Alison Lee
Edited by Mandy Greenfield, Claire Wedderburn-Maxwell
Consultant Editor: Marilyn Sherlock, MIT MAE, Chairman of the Institute of Trichologists

Reproduction by Global Colour, Malaysia
Printed and bound in Singapore by Imago

SAFETY NOTE
The information in this book is not intended as a substitute for medical advice. Any person suffering from conditions
requiring medical attention, or who has symptoms that concern them, should consult a qualified medical practictioner.

# CONTENTS

| | |
|---|---|
| Foreword | 6 |
| Hair: your crowning glory | 8 |
| | |
| HAIR STRUCTURE | 12 |
| Hair components | 14 |
| Patterns of growth | 16 |
| African Caribbean, Oriental and mixed-race hair | 20 |
| | |
| HAIR CARE | 22 |
| Introduction | 24 |
| Washing and shampooing | 26 |
| Drying hair | 38 |
| Brushing and combing | 40 |
| Hair products | 42 |
| Setting and styling | 44 |
| Cutting and holiday care | 46 |
| | |
| HAIR HEALTH | 48 |
| Health from the inside | 50 |
| All about trichologists | 56 |
| Alopecia | 58 |
| Hair loss treatments | 62 |
| Disorders of the scalp | 68 |

| | |
|---|---|
| Infections of the scalp | 70 |
| Dandruff | 72 |
| Unwanted hair | 74 |
| | |
| HAIR COLOUR | 78 |
| The range of colours | 80 |
| What causes hair colour? | 82 |
| Choosing a hair colour | 84 |
| Steps to a new colour | 92 |
| Highlights and lowlights | 98 |
| Colouring African Caribbean and grey hair | 100 |
| | |
| HAIR CUTS | 102 |
| Cutting your hair | 104 |
| Matching the shape of your face | 106 |
| Finding a good hairdresser | 108 |
| Hair cutting techniques and styles | 110 |
| Perming | 114 |
| | |
| Questions and answers | 122 |
| Index | 126 |

# FOREWORD

For at least 4,000 years people have been obsessed with their hair. The ancient Egyptians are known to have coloured their hair and adorned themselves with elaborate wigs, and 2,000 years later Julius Caesar wore laurel leaves around his head to camouflage his bald pate. Hair is still just as important to us today, which is strange, considering that we could all live quite healthily if we had no hair at all.

The fact is that hair is our means of identity – due to the wide range of hair colourings and haircuts, it can identify us as individuals and act as an expression of who we are. The hairstyle and shade that we choose reveal a great deal about ourselves, while the natural greying process ages us.

Due to research in cosmetology, trichology (the study of hair and its diseases) and medicine, we are now able to do whatever we please with our hair. If it is curly, we can straighten it; if it is blonde, we can make it dark. Some of the hair colouring methods used today are centuries old, while others are very new.

There is no doubt that when we lose our hair it causes distress, and for this reason people have over the centuries tried all sorts of remedies to prevent hair loss and to try to make hair grow. As a result, numerous myths have emerged and many so-called 'cures' have been produced. Our imagination appears to have no end, where hair loss is concerned. Fortunately, science has given us the opportunity to validate these claims and to establish how best to care for and nourish our hair, from both within and without.

Maggie Jones has also set out to do this in *Hair Secrets*. She has sifted out the misinformation and myth, leaving simply the facts and the reality. Almost daily, trichologists are asked questions such as 'What is dandruff?' and 'Why does hair fall out?' *Hair Secrets* answers these questions and many, many more.

*Marilyn Sherlock* MIT MAE
CHAIRMAN OF THE INSTITUTE OF TRICHOLOGISTS

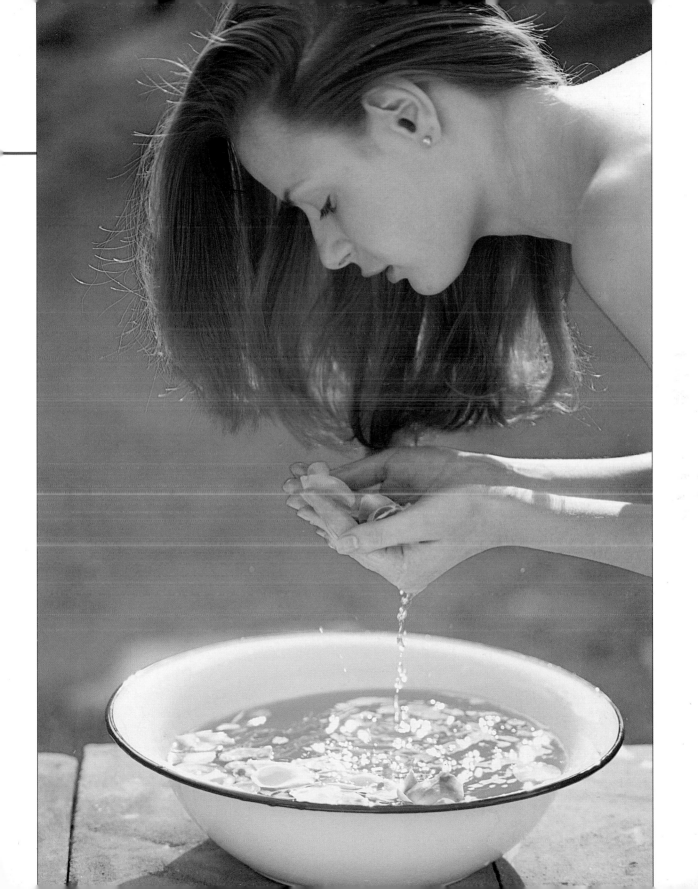

# Hair: YOUR
# CROWNING GLORY

**N**o single aspect of your looks will have as much initial impact as your hair – particularly for women. The style, colour, length and volume of your hair give a strong impression of your age, health and personality – and changing your hair dramatically can make you almost unrecognizable to those who don't know you well. How your hair looks and feels is so central to feeling good about yourself that the phrase 'bad hair day' has entered the language for those times when everything seems wrong about yourself and the world.

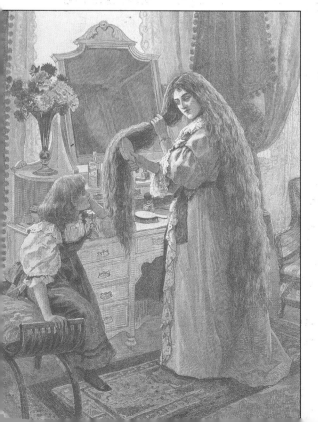

Most women would probably like to have long, thick, glossy, beautifully rich hair, like the models featured in hair advertisements, but may feel that this is impossible. Perhaps long hair would be too difficult to care for, or doesn't suit the shape of their head or face. Perhaps their hair is straight and very fine, without even the hint of a curl, or a dull, mousy colour, without any suggestion of a chestnut gleam? Many women would change all this, but hesitate to experiment with different hair colours, styles and treatments for fear that hair dyes and beauty products could end up damaging and spoiling their hair.

Women use a bewildering array of products on their hair – ordinary and medicated shampoos, conditioners, colourants, gels and sprays – without really knowing what works or what is best for their type of hair, or whether the products they are using clash with one another. Do frequent-wash shampoos really let you wash your hair twice a day without loosing its natural oils? Is conditioner really necessary every time? Do medicated shampoos for dandruff really work? The confusion is worsened by the fact that there is so much advertising of products, making sweeping claims about the effects they will have, without being backed up by any real, unbiased evidence.

While the number of hair products to condition, colour and beautify our hair has increased, there is evidence that beautiful hair is under attack from within the body, and that increased external levels of stress in the modern world have also affected our hair. More and more women are now complaining of hair loss, and excessive dieting and poor eating habits – a quick sandwich on the run – can prevent our hair being adequately nourished internally. Exposure to sun and pollutants, to chlorine in water and chemicals in the air can all damage hair; certain drugs and medications can also have adverse affects on its health and appearance.

This book aims to help you find out the facts about hair structure – how it grows and the different types of hair (see Chapter 1); how to keep your

hair healthy, how it is affected by your diet and lifestyle, and how you can nourish your hair from the inside (see Chapter 3). It will also give you information about the various hair-care treatments available, and what the active ingredients are in the shampoos, conditioners and colourants now available, including the new natural and organic products (see Chapter 2). It will help you to decide which products will best suit your hair and skin type and will suggest hair-care routines that are right for you.

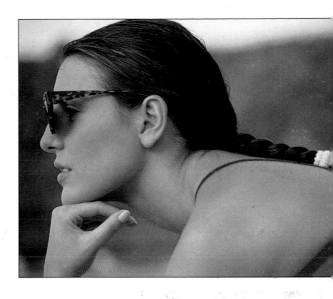

*Hair Secrets* will also show you how to make the best of your hair, to choose a cut and style that suits the shape of your face and head, your personality and your individual lifestyle (see Chapter 5). It will help you choose the colour that will go best with your skin tone, your age and the kind of clothes you like to wear (see Chapter 4), and it will find a hair-care routine that makes the most of your hair.

Rather than surrendering yourself passively to the hairdresser, asking, 'What can you do with my hair?' – or going to the other extreme and saying, 'I've always had my hair cut like this' – this book should enable you to develop your own ideas about what will suit you and what is possible, and how to sound knowledgeable and confident about your hair.

The book will also look at common hair problems, such as dry scalp, dandruff and split ends, and how to cure them (see Chapter 3). It will discuss normal hair loss and when this becomes a problem, and it offers advice about when and where you should go to seek further help.

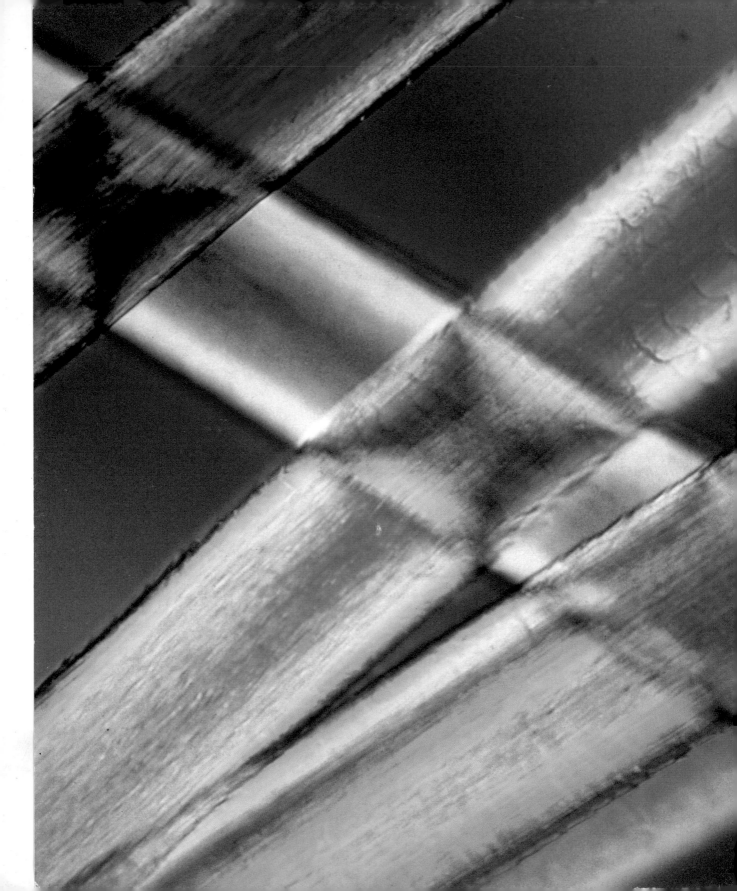

# HAIR
# Structure

# Hair COMPONENTS

Hair is formed from a down-growth in the skin. Each hair is made of a thin cylinder of keratin – a horny, elastic protein that is found in the cells and a softer version of which makes up the tough, outer layer of skin. Like the dead outer layer of skin cells, hairs contain neither blood vessels nor nerves.

Hair grows in hair follicles, which are tiny pits in the skin, about 4–7mm deep and 0.5mm wide. It grows continuously from the bulb at its base, which is sitting just above or in a layer of fat under the skin. It is nourished by blood vessels in the papilla, or projection, which extends into the hair bulb.

The bulb contains a group of cells that divide to produce the early hair shaft and keep dividing throughout the growth phase of the hair.

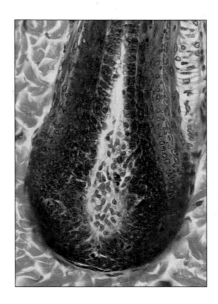

*Close-up of a hair follicle. The hair protrudes above the skin. At this point the hair is dead, although it continues to grow from the base.*

The keratin is laid down as the shaft matures and grows towards the mouth of the follicle.

The hair shaft is the part of the hair that protrudes above the skin. At this point the hair is dead and is made up of three layers: the cuticle, the cortex and the medulla (see diagram opposite).

## THE CUTICLE

This is made up of overlapping plates of keratin. It is more or less transparent, and the light shines through it to the natural colour within the hair shaft. The cuticle can be damaged by sunlight, chlorine and some hairdressing processes, such as bleaching and perming. It can also become damaged in old age or when the hair is long. When damaged, the cuticle lifts and hair becomes porous and dries out, making it likely to fray or split.

When the cuticle scales lie flat, the hair will feel soft and smooth and will look glossy. When they are damaged, the hair will be dull and brittle and will tangle easily.

## THE CORTEX

This layer, which makes up the bulk of the hair, contains fibres made of chains of amino acids twisted together called polypeptides. These chains are held together with chemical bonds, the strongest of which are known as disulphide bonds. These give hair its texture, elasticity, suppleness and strength. The cortex also contains the pigments (in cells called melanocytes) that give the hair its colour.

### THE MEDULLA

The medulla forms the central core of the hair, but it is not present in all hairs and only partially exists in some hairs. Where it is present, it is made up of spongy keratin with many air spaces. In the hair bulb, blood capillaries nourish the growing hair. Three main processes take place there: cell division, to make the hair grow; hair pigmentation, due to natural pigments being laid down in the hair cortex, and keratinization – the production of large quantities of the protein keratin.

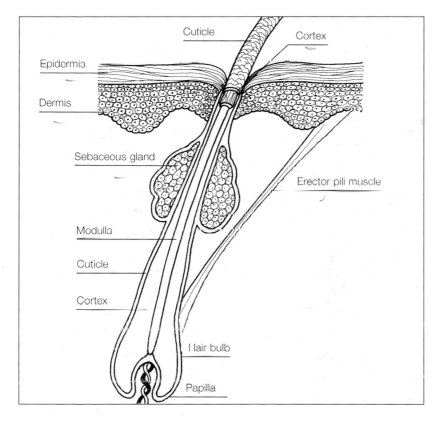

Cuticle
Cortex
Epidermis
Dermis
Sebaceous gland
Erector pili muscle
Modulla
Cuticle
Cortex
Hair bulb
Papilla

*Cross-section of the skin showing the hair follicle, with sebaceous gland and erector pili muscle.*

## Did you know?

| 1 | 2 | 3 | 4 | 5 | 6 |
|---|---|---|---|---|---|
| Each person has something like five million hair follicles all over their body. Only about 100,000 of these are found on the scalp. | Healthy hair is elastic and can stretch by 20 or 30 per cent of its length before snapping. | A human hair is actually stronger than the same thickness of copper wire. | A headful of human hair is so strong that it can support a weight equivalent to nearly 100 people. | You lose an average of 100 hairs from your scalp every day. | Your hair really does stand on end when you are scared. |

# Patterns OF GROWTH

Under the skin, the hair is held in place in the follicle by skin cells that interlock with the hair cuticle. These have cuticle scales, similar to those that are found on the outer hair shaft. Hairs are also locked in place by the chubby shape of the hair bulb. Sebaceous glands attached to the follicle produce the natural oil, known as sebum, that is released into the hair follicles; it coats the skin and hair shaft, smoothing the cuticle scales and keeping the hair waterproof and flexible. Sebum also acts as a mild antiseptic and helps reduce the risk of skin infections.

## HAIR DEVELOPMENT

In humans, the development of hair begins nine weeks after the egg has been fertilized. By the sixth month of pregnancy the foetus is covered by a growth of fine hair called lanugo hair. This is shed about one month before birth takes place. A second coat of lanugo hair is formed and then shed in all areas, except the scalp, during the first few months of life. This is in turn replaced by thick hair on the head and finer, downy hair on the body. The infant may be born with a thick head of hair, but this sometimes comes out, to be replaced with a different texture and colour of hair. On the other hand, some babies are born almost bald.

## PATTERNS OF GROWTH

The hair normally grows out of the skin at an angle, so that the fine body hairs tend to grow flat against the skin. On the scalp, the angle at which the follicles lie and the pattern of their distribution cause the natural direction of hair growth and create spontaneous partings and the formation of the crown. Attached to the hair follicle is a small bundle of smooth muscle that contracts to make the hair stand up when you are cold, or frightened or experiencing other powerful emotions.

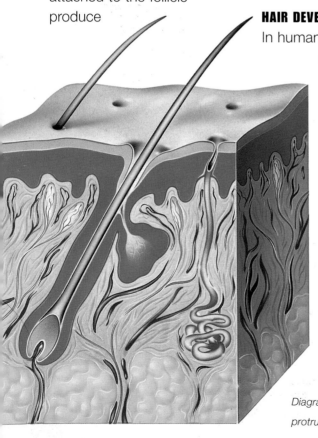

*Diagram showing a human hair protruding from the skin.*

## PATTERNS IN THE HAIR

Most of the hair on the head grows in the same direction – outwards, away from the crown – and this is determined by the angle of the hair follicles. However, patterns in hair growth may be caused by some hairs growing in a different direction. These include:

- A widow's peak, where the hair grows forward to form a V-shaped point in the centre of the forehead.

- A cowlick, or tuft of hair over the forehead, where the hair at the hairline grows in the opposite direction to the rest; this gives it the tendency to stand on end.

- A whorl, or loop, where the hair grows round in a circle, often at the crown of the head (sometimes there are two), although whorls can also occur at the nape of the neck.

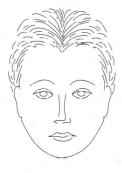

Widow's Peak

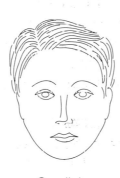

Cowlick

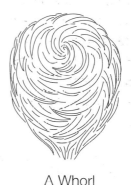

A Whorl

# TYPES OF HAIR

There are three main types of hair.

| | TYPE | LOCATION |
|---|---|---|
| 1 | Terminal hair | scalp, eyebrows, lashes, beard, pubic and underarm area |
| 2 | Vellus hair | fine downy hairs that grow all over the body, except where terminal hairs grow and on the palms of the hands and soles of the feet |
| 3 | Lanugo hair | fine hair in which newborn infants are covered before and at birth |

# THE CYCLE of hair growth

Each hair grows in a constant cycle and has a limited life. There are three phases in the life of a hair. First comes the active or anagen phase, in which the hair grows, usually at the rate of about 1.25cm ($^1/_2$in) each month, and which lasts for one to six years. This is followed by a short resting period or catagen phase lasting about two weeks, and then the hair is shed in the telogen phase, with new hair pushing up from underneath. Sometimes there can be more than one hair in a follicle, making for thicker, more luxuriant hair. About 100 scalp hairs are usually lost each day, to be replaced by new ones, so there is no need to worry when you see what looks like a lot of hair on your brush or comb, or in the sink after you wash your hair.

As you age, the growing phase gets shorter and the resting stage longer, so that it becomes difficult to grow your hair as long as it was in your youth. Hair density usually also reduces with age, although fewer women suffer from the pattern baldness that affects many men. Hair is at its thickest between the ages of 15 and 25; between 30 and 50 there is some thinning, but over the age of 50 – health and diet permitting – the hair should not thin much more. Far more noticeable than this thinning of hair is the loss of pigmentation, which usually starts around the age of 40, but sometimes much earlier, and leads ultimately to white hair. White hair is often drier and coarser, and usually has less sebum to coat, moisturize and protect it.

How curly or straight, thick or fine your hair is depends on the regularity of cell division at the base of the hair bulb. If the cells divide evenly, the hair will be straight. If they divide more rapidly on one side than on the other, then the hair will be curly. In African Caribbean hair, this growth is constantly corrected so that the hair bends first in one, then in another, direction, creating tight, crinkled curls.

While the curliness, texture and colour of our hair is genetically determined, with racial and individual differences, its texture can actually change over time. Hair often becomes curlier and greasier at adolescence, and frequently becomes drier after the menopause, although this may be associated with the effects of greying.

## HORMONAL CHANGES

During pregnancy hair may well become thicker. This is because the hair lives longer under the influence of higher levels of the female hormones, oestrogen and progesterone, that are produced in pregnancy. Much of the hair that would have been lost over these nine months is retained. Then, three months after the birth, these hairs fall out, with the hair reverting to its pre-pregnancy density. However, many women notice this extra hair loss and become alarmed. Hair will also fall out in the same way after an abortion or miscarriage.

Hair growth is different in men and women, and these differences emerge at puberty. Under the influence of the main sex hormones, women start to grow hair under their arms and in the pubic area. This hair, especially pubic hair, is usually thicker and curlier than the hair on the head. Pubic and underarm hair serves to trap the scent produced by special sweat glands in these areas, which is designed to be attractive to the opposite sex. In older women past the menopause, the pubic hair tends to thin out and become straighter. Eventually it may turn grey.

Unlike men, women do not normally develop long facial hair. Some women have more of the downy vellus hair than usual on their faces and, if the hair is very dark, this can be problematic. The development of thick, long facial hair is almost always the sign of a hormone imbalance or illness of some sort, as is the growth of thick, long hair elsewhere on the body.

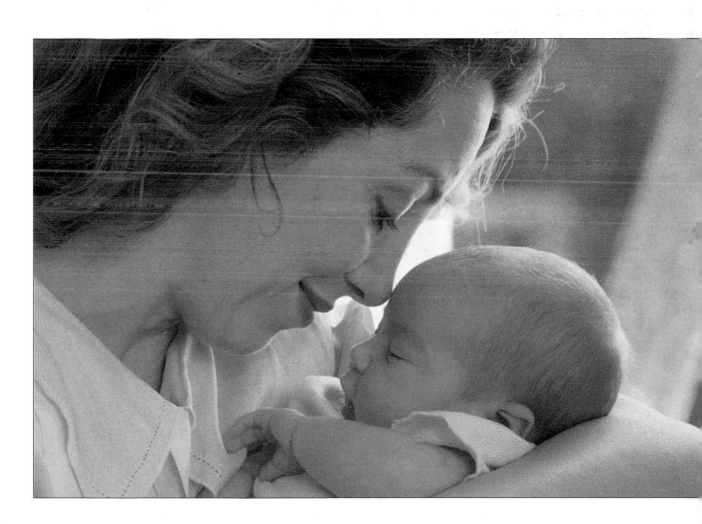

# African Caribbean, Oriental

# AND MIXED-RACE HAIR

**A**frican and African Caribbean hair has a different texture and shape from European (Caucasian) hair, being elliptical in cross-section, rather than oval. While wavy European hair curls in one direction, African Caribbean hair curls both around and along its axis, in different directions at various points in the hair. The texture also varies along the hair shaft, making it more porous in some places than in others. This can cause problems when hair products are applied, as the hair may take up the chemicals unevenly.

The cuticle of African Caribbean hair has seven to eleven layers, compared with the four to seven layers of European hair. Its twisting nature prevents the layers of the cuticle lying flat, and this means that less light is reflected from the hair, making it duller in appearance. The tight curl in African Caribbean hair results from two types of cortex: the ortho-cortex on the outside of the curl and the para-cortex on the inside (the para-cortex is more dense than the ortho-cortex). Unlike Caucasian hair, the pigment is contained in the cuticle and the medulla, as well as in the cortex. The granules of pigment are also larger than those found in European hair.

Some people have written that African Caribbean hair may grow more slowly than European hair, but in fact this is not usually the case. The hair appears shorter because the dense curl does not allow it to fall to the same extent, and it also has a shorter life. The growth stage of this type of hair may last for as little as nine or ten months – but more usually for around two years – so that it simply does not grow as long: 20cm (8in) is quite long for African Caribbean hair.

It is important when plaiting this kind of hair not to put too much tension into the hair at the roots, as this can cause traction alopecia (see p.61). Chemically treated hair should be conditioned before plaiting, and all hair should be shampooed first. Cornrowed hair should be shampooed once a week at the roots only, leaving the plaits and beads untouched.

African Caribbean hair may become very dry and brittle, due to the climate, and needs special care. Conditioners, oils and waxes containing protein, lanolin and natural and mineral oils are often applied to it to counteract these drying influences.

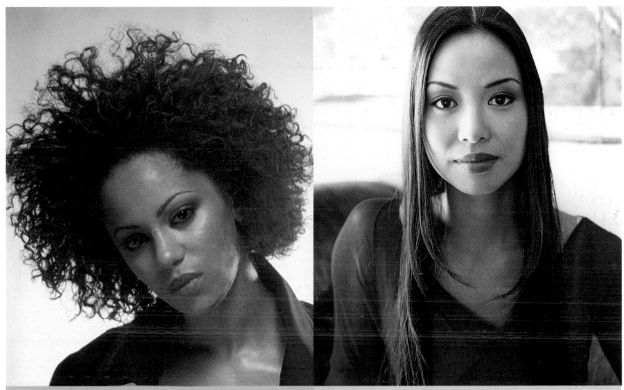

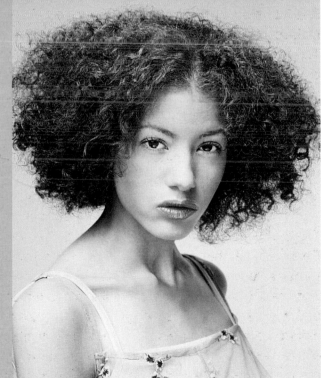

Black hair can be intensely curly, while Oriental hair is strong and straight. Oriental hair is also round in cross-section, has eleven or more layers of cuticle, and lives for a long time, so many Oriental women can grow their hair right down to the ground. People of mixed race may have a combination of different types of hair on the same head, which creates its own special requirements for care.

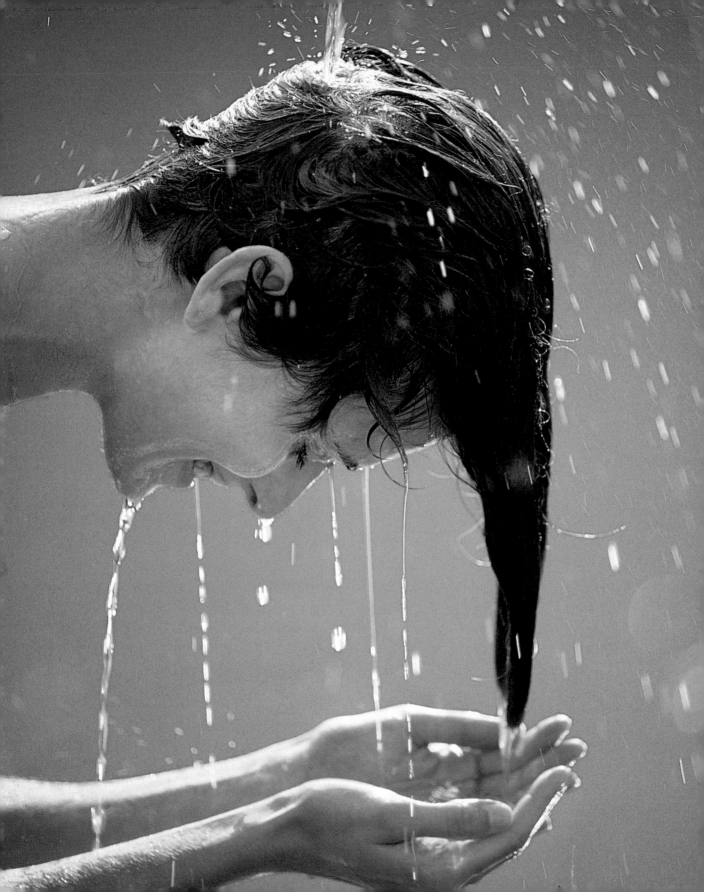

# HAIR
# Care

# INTRODUCTION

How you care for your hair will depend on its texture; whether it is dry, normal or greasy; and whether it has been chemically treated – bleached, dyed or permed. There are three main elements in hair care: cleaning or shampooing; conditioning; and brushing or combing. In addition, you may need to protect your hair from the sun or from chlorine and other chemicals.

Today there is a bewildering number of hair products to choose from, and very little advice on which ones would best suit your hair. By looking at what many of these products actually contain – and which ingredients are active – you will be able to make a more realistic choice.

A thick head of glowing, healthy hair is what we all seek, but it is not always clear how to achieve it.

Some people advise washing your hair less often, to preserve the natural oils; others washing your hair every day. Washing out natural oils and replacing them with artificial ones in the form of conditioners sounds stupid, but this is what most of us have to do to keep our hair clean and in good shape. Diet, too, can be important in nourishing the hair and giving it bounce and shine. Your general health and the health of your skin can likewise have an effect on the appearance of your hair.

Before you begin, it is important to establish your hair type and exactly what kind of hair routine will best suit you. You can then work out what kind of shampoo and conditioner to use, how best to brush, comb and dry it, and how to use the many different kinds of applications and hair-care aids.

## DIFFERENT TYPES OF HAIR
### Dry hair
Dry hair looks dull, and may tangle easily, in which case it will be difficult to comb or brush. It is also more likely to split at the ends. Dryness may be the natural state of your hair, due to your hair follicles tending to produce too little sebum or natural oils. Excessive shampooing, misuse of colours or perms, damage from the sun or harsh weather conditions can also dry your hair.

### Normal hair
Normal hair is neither greasy nor dry and looks good most of the time. It is easy to care for and doesn't require much effort to keep it looking healthy and shining.

### Greasy hair
Greasy hair, by contrast, looks lank and oily. This is caused by an over-production of sebum, which may be

linked to hormonal disturbances, stress, or a diet too rich in saturated fat, but is more commonly genetically inherited. Greasy hair also becomes dirty more quickly than other hair types, as it attracts more dust and dirt.

## Combination hair

This hair type is greasy at the roots, but often dry and sometimes split at the ends, when shampooed too often or with the wrong shampoo. It frequently occurs in hair that has been harshly treated with chemicals and over-strong shampoos, or that has been over-exposed to sunlight and heating and setting equipment. The scalp produces too much sebum, while the ends are damaged and lose moisture.

## Coloured or permed hair

Hair that has been coloured or permed is frequently more fragile and porous than untreated hair. The colour may fade and the hair may become brittle.

## Afro hair

A wide variety of products is made especially for use on African Caribbean hair. This hair can be more difficult to shampoo than other hair, because the tight curl makes it so dense. More shampoo may be needed and great care must be taken to rinse the hair thoroughly. Due to the dressings on the hair, it is sometimes useful to apply the shampoo to dry hair, adding the water slowly to produce a lather.

Shampoos that are acidic are best for use on Afro hair, as these tangle less easily. This should be followed by a conditioning product, perhaps with a hydrolized keratin conditioner, which will lower the hair's porosity, make it easier to handle and attract moisture into the cortex. Many shampoos are also conditioning, using oils such as almond, coconut or olive to help overcome the tendency to dryness.

Conditioners for African Caribbean hair may also contain silicones, which leave behind a film of protective polymer after rinsing. Many products also contain lanolin, the natural sebum produced by sheep, and special moisturizers are available.

Wide-toothed combs are best for gently untangling the hair; work through it gradually in sections. Do not comb the hair when it is wet, as it is liable to damage. Allowing the hair to dry naturally rather than using a hairdrier will help conserve moisture.

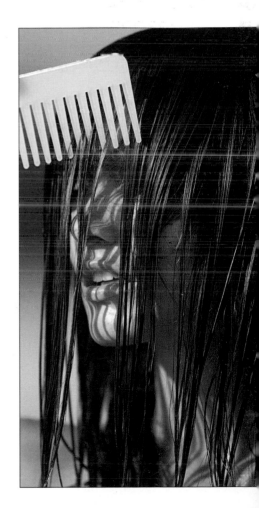

# Washing
# AND SHAMPOOING

The first and most important consideration in caring for the hair is keeping it clean. The hair will inevitably be made dirty by skin flakes, salt from dried sweat, and dust and dirt in the environment. While these alone would wash off easily enough, they become mixed with the oily sebum that coats the scalp and hair shaft. This combination does not easily dissolve in water, so water by itself is not enough to clean your hair.

The skin on the scalp also has small pits and wrinkles, while the surface of the hair shaft is not smooth (as the scales of the cuticle overlap), thereby leaving small spaces where dirt can lodge. Water alone is unable to penetrate these areas, as it is repelled by the layer of oil, so you will also need to add a soapless detergent.

Although water needs to penetrate the hair to reach all the dirt, the cleaning agent must not be so harsh that it removes all the sebum from the hair and scalp. This would leave the hair dry and the scalp vulnerable to infection, especially since the sebum contains a natural antiseptic. Anything used to clean the hair must therefore be strong enough to lift off the dirt, but not so strong that it damages the hair. It should also leave the hair in good condition.

## SHAMPOO: WHAT'S IN IT?

Modern shampoos have been developed to clean the hair efficiently but gently. Shampoos contain a soapless detergent that reduces the surface tension of the water and enables the water molecules to reach the small crevices in the skin and hair.

The detergent also emulsifies the oil, breaking it into tiny droplets that can then be washed away by the water. The detergent molecules surround the dirt particles, preventing them being redeposited on the hair.

## MAIN INGREDIENTS

Shampoos contain a wide range of ingredients to suit different types and conditions of hair. The main ingredient is the detergent, also known as a surfactant (short for surface-active agent).

The majority of shampoos use sodium or ammonium lauryl sulphates as the principal surfactant. These have the strongest lathering and cleansing properties, but can occasionally irritate the scalp. Laureth sulphates are slightly more gentle and less irritant, and give greater shine to the hair.

Secondary surfactants are added to the shampoo to help to maintain a rich lather, increase the efficiency of the main detergent, improve the condition of the hair and reduce the possibility of irritation of the scalp. They include alkyl phosphates, methyl taurides, fatty-acid alkanolamides, acyl amino acids, sarcosines and peptides. The gentlest are alkyl amino acids, betains and alkyl imidazoline compounds.

*The most common preservatives used in shampoos are the parabens, formaldehyde, Bronidox and methyl chloroisothiazolinones (Kathon CG). Anyone with a scalp disorder should avoid formaldehyde, as this is more likely than the other preservatives to sensitize the skin.*

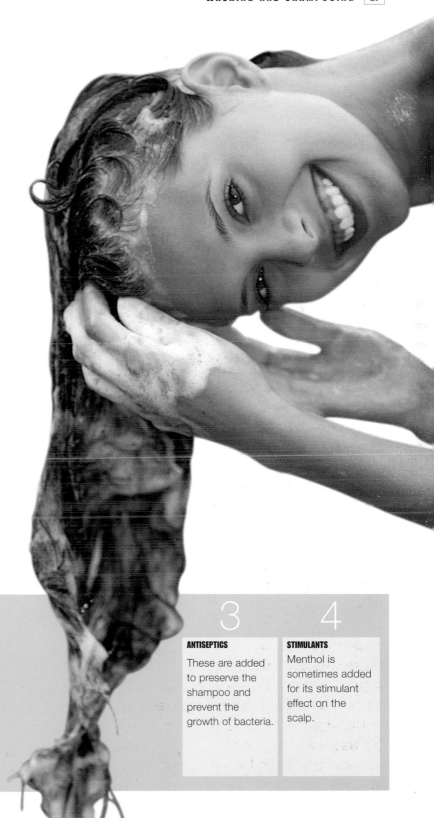

# Other ingredients:

## 1
**COMMON SALT**
This is added to thicken the shampoo and can be found in most types of shampoo.

## 2
**ACIDS (E.G. CITRUS ACID)**
This conditions the hair by leaving it slightly acid after shampooing. Often found in 'pH balance' or 'acid balance' shampoos.

## 3
**ANTISEPTICS**
These are added to preserve the shampoo and prevent the growth of bacteria.

## 4
**STIMULANTS**
Menthol is sometimes added for its stimulant effect on the scalp.

# SHAMPOO additives

A range of additional ingredients may be added to shampoos and should be selected for their effects on the hair.

## PROTEINS

Many shampoos are advertised as protein shampoos. They are often obtained from protein substances – soya is a common example, and egg may also be added. The manufacturers suggest that the proteins will adhere to the porous regions of the hair. While this may be the case, the surest way to add protein to the hair is to eat protein foods, as this helps the hair to form correctly in the first place.

## BEER

This is sometimes added to shampoos: the beer coats each hair, thickening it slightly and adding body and shine to the whole head.

## FRUITS

Extracts of fruit, in the form of fruit sugars, are sometimes used in shampoos, as they draw in moisture from the air and hydrate the hair.

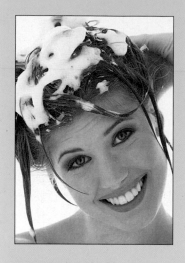

**LABEL SHOWING TYPICAL SHAMPOO INGREDIENTS:**

INGREDIENTS  Aqua, Ammonium Laureth Sulfate, Glycol Distearate, Sodium Chloride, Sodium Citrate, Cocamide MEA, Dimethicone, Panthenyl Ethyl Ether, Cetyl Alcohol, Stearyl Alcohol, Sodium Benzoate, Citric Acid, Ammonium Xylenesulfonate, DMDM Hydantoin, Tetrasodium EDTA, Parfum.

**SYNTHETIC CHEMICALS** *used directly on the hair and skin have long been a source of concern. If you take care with what you eat and how you exercise, it makes sense to think about what you apply externally, too. The text on page 30 offers a guide to what the specific chemicals you see on your hair product packaging actually do.*

*Any chemicals that strip the hair of its colour – typically those listed as sulphides and oxides – are causing some damage to the surface of the hair. Many of the shampoos and conditioners that come as part of a colourant contain ingredients specifically devised to counteract this damage; always use the whole pack.*

# HERBS

Many herbs are used in shampoos and other hair preparations as they contain natural substances that have different effects on the hair. You need to choose a preparation that will suit the texture and colour of your hair.

| | | |
|---|---|---|
| 1 | Rosemary | Has antiseptic properties and can be used to treat dandruff and other scalp problems. |
| 2 | Juniper | May stimulate hair growth and acts as a strong antiseptic. |
| 3 | Cedarwood | Can help an itchy or flaky scalp. |
| 4 | Tea tree | The oil can help with an itchy scalp or dandruff. |
| 5 | Chamomile | Has a drying effect on greasy hair and is used to add highlights to fair hair. |
| 6 | Lemongrass | Also used to treat greasy hair. |
| 7 | Almond | Contains proteins and amino acids that help thicken fine hair. |
| 8 | Aloe vera | Acts as a general hair tonic. |
| 9 | Comfrey | Can be used to treat dry hair. |
| 10 | Lavender | Can be used to treat oily hair. |
| 11 | Nettle | Extract of nettle root is used for oily hair. |
| 12 | Ginger root | Acts as an astringent and is used in some shampoos to treat dandruff; it is claimed to nourish the skin when taken by mouth. |
| 13 | Coconut | For moisturizing dry hair. |
| 14 | Macassar | Indian macassar oil is rich in oleic and linoleic acid and is used for dry, dehydrated and brittle hair. |
| 15 | Safflower | Safflower seed is rich in fatty acids and the oil can be used on damaged or brittle hair. |

# OTHER shampoo additives

Other ingredients may also be added to shampoos to help protect against dandruff or the harmful effects of chlorine, or to bleach the hair.

### BLEACHES
Sometimes a small amount of hydrogen peroxide is added to shampoo as a mild bleach.

### ANTI-DANDRUFF AGENTS
Scaling or flaking of the scalp is sometimes caused by bacteria. Anti-bacterial ingredients, such as cetrimide BP or phenethyl alcohol, are added to some shampoos in order to treat this. Fungal infections may also cause dandruff. If this is a problem for you, then use a shampoo to which anti-fungal ingredients have been added; the most common is undecenoic acid BP.

To slow down cell growth in the germinative layer of the epidermis (the outer layer of the skin), selenium sulphide or zinc pyrithione are used. The former should not be used within 48 hours of tinting or perming the hair,

or there may be a reaction between this substance and the ammonium compounds in tints and perms.

Irritation and scaling of the scalp are often assisted by the use of coal-tar products, as these are antiseptic and lessen irritation. For cases where the scalp is simply dry, coconut fatty acids are added, and fruit sugars may help to moisturize the scalp as well as the hair. Urea may also be used to add body to limp hair.

### ANTI-CHLORINE AGENTS
Some shampoos have been formulated to undo the harmful effects of chlorine in swimming pools. These often contain a substance called EDTA, which attaches itself to chlorine and to the metal ions, removing them from the hair. This will prevent discoloration of the hair by these metals.

### WATCH OUT FOR:
- Harsh surfactants that remove every trace of sebum from the scalp.

- Irritation of the scalp and eyes after shampooing – if you experience this, use another shampoo.

- Highly perfumed and coloured shampoos. Perfumes and colours are added to shampoos to make them pleasant to use and a recognizable product. Nearly all sensitization reactions to shampoos are due to either the perfume or the preservative. This happens very rarely, however, because most products are in contact with the scalp for only a short time. Occasionally irritation may result when the shampoo is not completely rinsed away after use.

### FINDING THE RIGHT SHAMPOO
Always use the correct kind of shampoo for your hair type. Look at the label – most will specify what type of hair they are designed for.

Test different shampoos to find one that is right for you – try small sachets or samples.

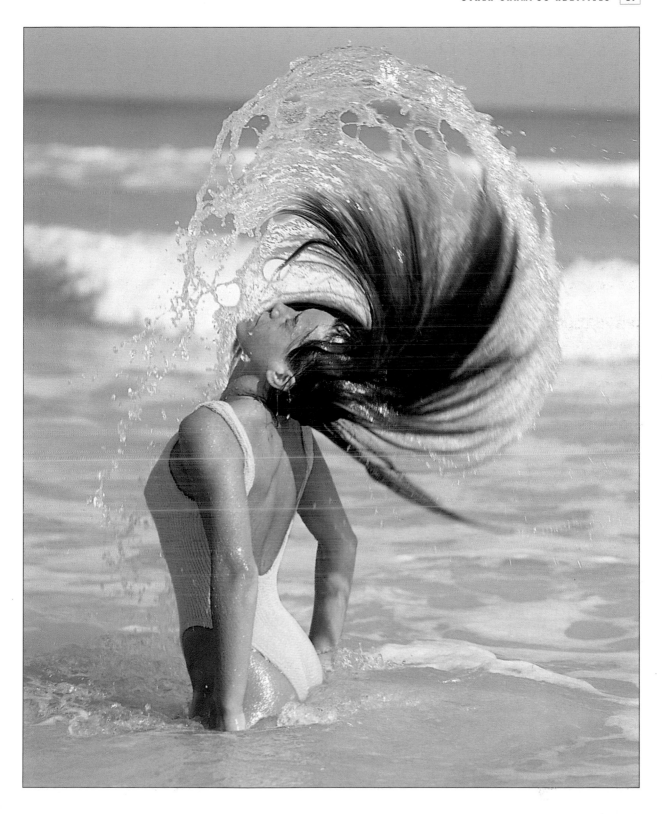

# SHAMPOO: how to use it

Soap is unsuitable for use on hair as it is too harsh and also leaves a sticky deposit on the hair, especially in hard water areas. Modern shampoos use soapless detergents that leave the hair clean and shiny. There are a large number of brands and types of shampoo available, so shop around to find a shampoo that suits your hair.

## HOW OFTEN SHOULD YOU SHAMPOO?

How often you wash your hair will depend on your lifestyle and how dirty it gets, plus the type of hair you have – dry, normal or greasy.

As a rule, greasy hair needs shampooing more often than dry hair. The most important thing, however, is the level of dirt your hair is exposed to. If you live and work in the city, travel on buses, underground trains or by rail, or work in an environment that is polluted, you will have to wash your hair frequently. If so, you should take care to replace the lost oils with conditioner.

Some people believe that hair should not be washed too frequently because this removes too much oil from the hair. This is an idea derived from the days when the air was cleaner, and shampoos as we know them had yet to be invented, but it does not apply today. With modern shampoos and pollution levels, hair needs regular washing. If the dirt builds up, it can damage the hair and scalp and become more difficult to remove.

Frequent washing – provided a mild shampoo is used, which strips less of the sebum from the hair, and is followed each time by a conditioner – should not harm the hair. Even washing the hair as often as once a day should not be damaging to it.

A build-up of hair products normally causes a problem only if the hair is very porous, due to being overtreated, coloured or permed, or on very long and therefore old hair, where it may adhere more and make the hair feel

tacky. Hairdressers may have a problem in tinting or perming, since the hair may be protected to some degree from the chemicals being used. In this case, shampoos that simply clean the hair (and do not condition it) are best.

## THE PH FACTOR

pH (short for potential of hydrogen) is used as a measure of acidity and alkalinity. Sebum naturally has a pH of between 4.5 (which is mildly acidic) and 7 ( which is neutral). Bacteria do not thrive in this environment. Many shampoos are therefore formulated to have a pH that is roughly the same as sebum, to help keep bacteria down and protect the hair.

## WHICH SHAMPOO?

It is sometimes claimed that it is best to alternate the shampoo you use, but there is no evidence that using only one shampoo will harm your hair, unless you have chosen the wrong type of shampoo in the first place. '

# THE SHAMPOOING PROCESS

Telling someone how to shampoo their hair sounds a bit like teaching your grandmother to suck eggs, but many people shampoo without thinking, following instructions they were given years ago, such as always having to use two lots of shampoo, or applying too much or too little shampoo. There are also many old wives' tales about washing hair – such as the one that washing hair in cold water increases its shine.

1 Always read the instructions on the bottle first – some shampoos recommend that you leave them on for a few minutes before rinsing.

2 Soak the hair thoroughly in warm water, as sebum will not dissolve in cold water.

3 Use a small dollop of shampoo on short hair, a medium dollop on longer hair, and spread it between your hands to ensure an even spread before stroking it through your hair.

4 Pay special attention to the hairline area, as this is where dirt and old make-up can lodge.

5 Gently massage the shampoo into the roots of the hair with the tips of your fingers – never your nails.

6 Rinse the hair thoroughly, as any residue left on it may cause the cuticle to break down or become more porous.

7 Only if your hair was very dirty or the product did not lather well the first time do you need to shampoo it again.

8 Rinse your hair in clean, warm water – don't rinse it in the bathwater, as soap residue will cling to the hair and make it dull and porous.

9 Rinse several times until the water runs clear.

10 Blot the hair dry with a clean towel. Too much vigorous rubbing of wet hair can stretch and damage it.

11 Long hair is best shampooed under a shower, as it minimizes the tangling that often results when hair is shampooed leaning forwards over a basin. The back-wash basins used in most hair salons work in the same way as the shower.

# CONDITIONERS

Conditioners are usually acidic and may be oil- or wax-based substances that are applied to the hair to replace some of the oils lost during shampooing.

It may seem absurd to wash the protective sebum out of the hair and then replace it with other substances. However, dirt, chemicals and other pollutants cling to the sebum that coats the hair shaft and scalp, and they need to be regularly removed. Conditioners are then necessary to restore the lost moisture and to create a glossy shine.

## TYPES OF CONDITIONER

There are three main types of conditioner: basic, oil-based conditioners; 'substantive' conditioners, which add material to the hair; and acid-type conditioners.

## BASIC CONDITIONERS

These are normally oils suspended in an emulsion of water to make a creamy substance that is easy to apply to the hair. Lanolin, from sheep's wool, is often used as a substitute for sebum.

## SUBSTANTIVE CONDITIONERS

These become fixed to, or absorbed into, the hair shaft, coating the hair. As well as the conditioning agent, they include some soapless detergents and polyvinyl pyrrolidone (PVP), which acts both as a setting agent and as a conditioner.

## ACID CONDITIONERS

These are used to restore the natural, slightly acidic pH of the hair. They can be used to neutralize alkaline deposits left on the hair after perming, bleaching or tinting. They may also be applied to make sure that the final pH of the hair is acidic. Organic acids, such as citric acid, tartaric acid and lactic acid, are often used.

These three basic types of conditioner are packaged in many different ways to make a variety of treatments. These include:

## HOT OILS

These can be used for a deep conditioning treatment. They usually come in a tube that can be placed in hot water for a minute or so before applying the oil.

The hair should be wetted, dabbed dry with a towel, and the hot oil should be massaged evenly into the hair and scalp. The head can then be covered with a shower cap. The oils are left on for a specified period, then shampooed and rinsed away.

## HENNA WAX CONDITIONERS

These thick, colourless products are used for a deep conditioning treatment. They are applied in the same way as hot oils and have no effect on hair colour.

## CONDITIONING SPRAYS

These may be used before styling the hair, as they protect it against the harmful effects of heat when the hair is dried. They can also reduce static on fine or flyaway hair.

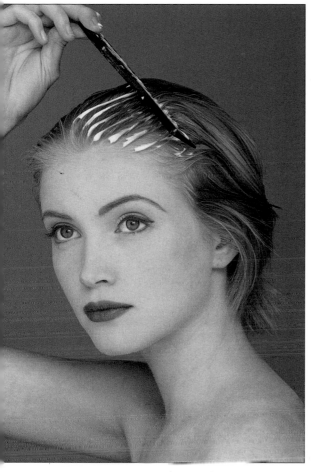

and add shine. They are used mainly on very dry, damaged or flyaway hair. Some are designed to be used daily.

## RESTRUCTURANTS

These contain proteins that may be deposited on the cuticle or even absorbed into the cortex in areas where the hair is damaged, thus temporarily strengthening it.

They are usually recommended for hair that has been damaged by excessive treatments, although they may in fact be of more use in protecting hair against damage. Remember that badly damaged hair cannot be repaired, although these conditioners will help it to remain supple for longer than it otherwise would.

## AFTER-COLOUR AND AFTER-PERM CONDITIONERS

After-colour conditioners add a protective film around the porous areas of treated hair, which can prevent colour loss. After-perm products help stabilize the hair, restoring the correct pH balance and helping it to keep its curl and bounce.

## SPLIT-END TREATMENTS

These are designed for damaged hair. They surround it with a microscopic film, which makes the hair shaft smoother and more shiny. The 'repair' to the split ends lasts only until the next shampoo, or until brushing and combing remove it, and is not permanent.

## SUN-BLOCK CONDITIONERS

Some conditioners are formulated with an ultraviolet screen to protect the hair against the harmful effects of the sun.

## INTENSIVE CONDITIONERS

These are designed to help the hair replenish its natural elasticity and condition. They are applied evenly to wet hair after shampooing and are left on for 5, 10, 15 or even 20 minutes, then rinsed out well in fresh water.

## LEAVE-IN CONDITIONERS

These can be left on the hair after shampooing to help retain moisture, reduce static

# SCALP massage

Massage helps to maintain a healthy scalp by improving the circulation of blood, which delivers nutrients and oxygen to the hair follicle. It is best avoided if the hair is excessively oily, however, as it increases sebum production. It can also help to loosen dead skin cells from the scalp. Massage of the neck and shoulders also relaxes the neck muscles, which, when tense, can cut down on the free circulation of blood to the hair and scalp.

It is ideal if someone else can massage your scalp for you, either at a hair salon or at home. However, you can easily learn the right technique and massage your own hair every time you shampoo. There are three main kinds of massage: effleurage, petrissage and friction.

## EFFLEURAGE

This is a stroking movement applied to the scalp with the fingers in a slow, rhythmic manner. It can be used to relieve tension and relax the muscles.

Both hands are held at the centre front of the head and then pulled firmly down the back to the nape of the neck. The hands are then placed at either side of the temples and pulled firmly back round the contours at the side of the head, down to the neck and then on to the shoulders.

This kind of massage is best performed by someone else; teach your partner or family how to do this for you.

## PETRISSAGE

This is a slow, firm, kneading movement in which the skin is rotated over the skull bones underneath the fingers. It increases blood circulation and stimulates the glands and muscles.

The fingers are placed well spread out on the scalp and the skin is then rotated over the skull, without the fingers sliding over the scalp. The right hand moves in a clockwise direction while the left hand moves in an anti-clockwise direction.

The hands are lifted from their position and moved to new areas until the whole scalp has been massaged. Begin in the nape of the neck, work around the ears to the front hairline, then back across the top of the head, ending at the nape. Leave one hand in place while moving the other, as this makes the massage more continuous and pleasant. This is easy to do yourself while shampooing or conditioning your hair.

## FRICTION

This is the more familiar massage that many people use when washing their hair. The fingers are directed in quick, vigorous movements over the scalp.

It helps to start at the front of the head, then move the fingers firmly over the scalp in circular movements down to the nape of the neck, and back again.

A head massage should leave you with a feeling of relaxation, invigoration and well-being.

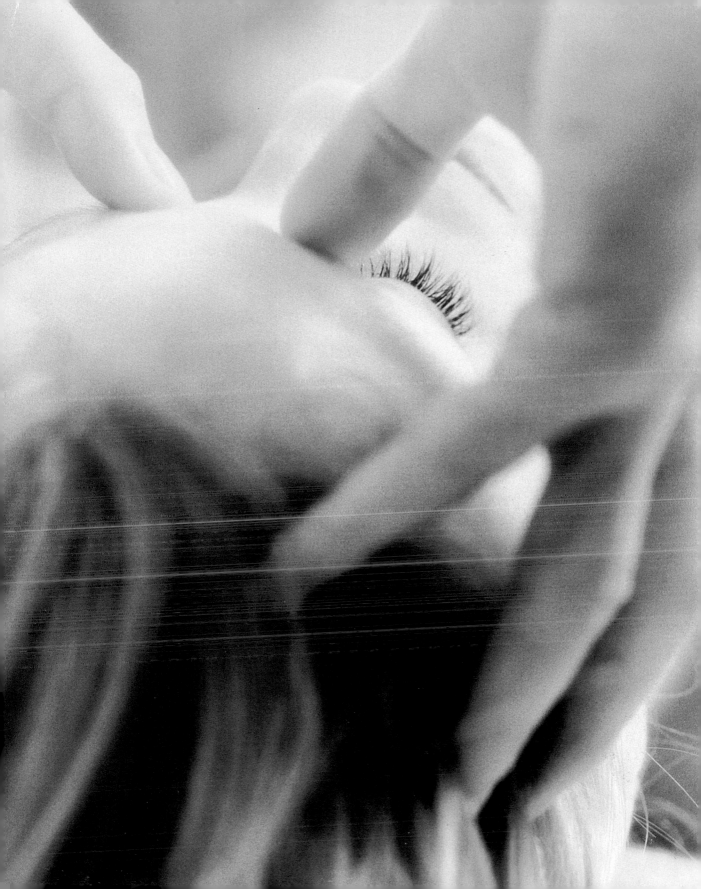

# Drying HAIR

The best way to dry the hair is to let it dry naturally. The hair may be dabbed dry with a towel – over-vigorous rubbing can damage the hair, especially if it is fragile – and then left to dry slowly in the air. This will retain the maximum amount of moisture, and natural drying will tend to keep long, straight hair sleek and will usually allow curly hair to wave naturally.

Many people, however, do not have time to allow their hair to dry naturally, especially if it is thick or long, or if they have to go straight to work after washing, or go straight to bed. The easiest way to dry the hair is with a small, hand-held blow-drier. However, always remember that overheating can dry out and damage the hair.

You can encourage the hair to curl when blow-drying it by winding the hair around a brush and holding it in place in the jet of hot air, or by using a diffuser. Blow-drying

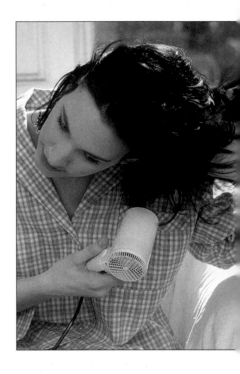

## Tips for using hairdriers:

| 1 | 2 | 3 | 4 | 5 | 6 |
|---|---|---|---|---|---|
| Do not hold the hairdrier too close to the hair, as this can cause it to overheat and cut out as well as damaging the hair. | Have the hairdrier on the lowest possible setting that will still have a good drying effect. | Start with the drier on a higher setting, when the hair is very wet, and reduce the heat to finish off the drying process. | The jet of air should follow the direction of the hair. Pointing the hairdrier in the opposite direction will ruffle the cuticle. | Never allow the jet of air to blow directly on to the scalp, as this can dry out or even damage it. | Keep the drier moving constantly to prevent the hair from overheating. |

the hair with the head upside-down can create lift and body. Alternatively, for a smooth, sleek look, comb the hair straight when drying.

Finger-drying works well for short, spiky or curly hair. The action of the fingers will help the hair to stand up or curl, and the fingers are gentler on the hair than a comb or brush. You can also carry out a friction massage of the scalp at the same time.

## CHOOSING A HAIRDRIER

Hairdriers will get a great deal of use, so select one carefully. A good hairdrier will have a range of settings for hot, medium and cool air and different speed settings, too. A diffuser is fitted to the nozzle to dry curly hair. The idea is that the diffuser spreads the air-flow over the hair, so that the curls are not literally blown away.

Choose a hairdrier with the potential for high power, but of the lightest weight available. This makes blow-drying, with your hands held above your head for approximately 15 minutes, much easier.

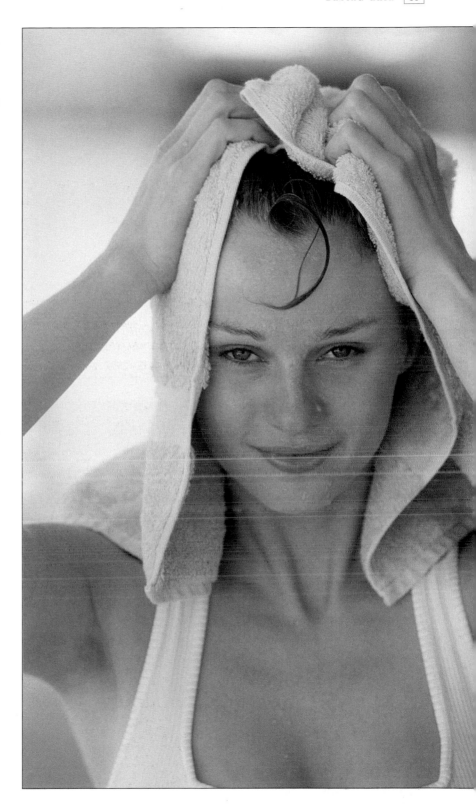

# Brushing
## AND COMBING

Brushing helps loosen knots and untangle the hair, and the action can loosen dead cells from the scalp and stimulate the circulation of the blood. The action of brushing from the roots to the tips also helps smooth the cuticle and makes the hair shine.

Hair should always be brushed when dry, never when wet, when it can easily be stretched or damaged. If you have long hair that tends to tangle easily, brushing is best done before washing and shampooing. To remove tangles and knots, start by using a wide-toothed comb, then move on to a brush, starting at the tips of the hair and working your way back towards the roots.

While a quick brush or a run of a comb through the hair can help make it look good, too much brushing and combing can actually harm it, especially if the hair is already dry or damaged. When combing or brushing is too vigorous, the mechanical scraping of the teeth of the comb or the bristles of the brush roughen the cuticle. With backcombing or backbrushing, the brushing action goes from the tip of the hair towards the root, rubbing the cuticle in the wrong direction and making the scales stand up rather than lie down. This leaves the hair looking dull and may make it liable to further damage. The increased friction caused by brushing and combing can also create static electricity, which makes the hair stand up and gives it a 'flyaway' look.

Historically, brushing the hair was necessary because it was washed much less often. The hair was therefore greasier or oilier, and brushing and combing enabled the sebum to be spread more evenly throughout the hair, acting as a natural conditioner; the sebum could also be brushed from the hair, taking the dirt with it. Nowadays, when hair is washed so frequently, such regular, vigorous brushing is no longer necessary.

Wide-toothed combs can be used when the hair is wet, and are also useful for spreading conditioner into the hair. They are essential if your hair is long.

### BRUSHES
Brushes may be made of natural bristles (usually hog's hair) or from plastic, nylon or wire. The bristles are embedded in a wooden, plastic or moulded base and are usually set in rows or tufts, allowing loose hairs to

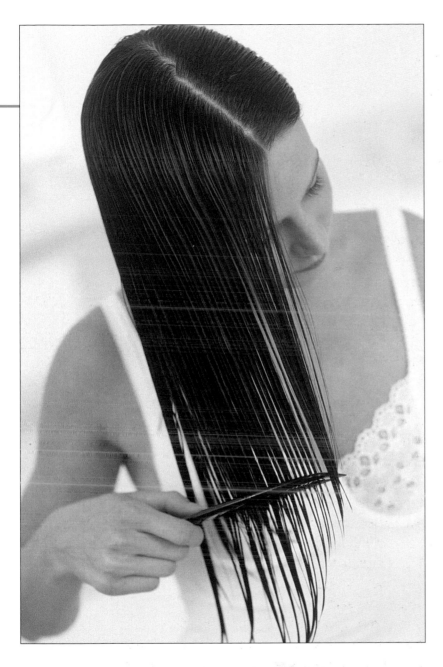

Natural bristle brushes should be allowed to dry naturally. If you use a pneumatic brush with a rubber-cushion base, the air-hole should be blocked before washing.

Finding the right brush is important. The best ones are cushioned, as these give flexibility as they glide through the hair, thus preventing tugging. Very rigid brushes are not ideal, because if the brush hits a tangle and will not give, then the hair will tear.

Natural bristle brushes are preferable to plastic ones if you suffer from problems with static electricity in the hair. Try to find plastic brushes with rounded tips; brushes with small balls at the tip may be more gentle on the scalp, but they can catch in your hair, especially if it is curly and tends to tangle or knot.

## COMBS

Good-quality combs have teeth that are individually cut into the comb, so that there are no sharp edges. Wide-toothed combs are recommended for use on very curly or African Caribbean hair.

collect in the grooves without interfering with the action of the bristles. The wider the spaces between the rows, the more easily the brush will slip through the hair.

Brushes should be cleaned once a week by pulling out the dead hairs and washing the base and bristles in warm, soapy water before drying them thoroughly.

# Hair PRODUCTS

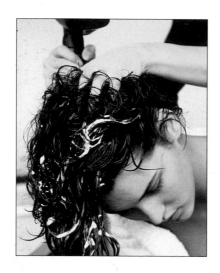

There is a wide range of different products – creams, waxes, sprays, shine enhancers – to choose from to enhance and hold the hair in the style that you choose.

### DRESSING CREAMS, SHINE ENHANCERS AND WAXES

These are used to reduce static electricity and to replace the natural oils lost in shampooing. Most dressing creams are made from mineral oil with perfume added. Mineral oils are preferred to vegetable oils, because they do not go rancid and they stay on the surface of the hair rather than penetrating the hair shaft, thereby producing more shine. Vegetable oils may, however, be more acceptable on sensitive skins. Animal oils, such as lanolin, are also used.

Only a small amount of cream is needed. Place a dollop about the size of a pea in your palm, then rub the palms together before stroking the hair with your hands, taking care not to forget the underneath layers. Do not use too much dressing cream or the hair will appear greasy and lank. Brush the hair afterwards to distribute the cream evenly throughout the hair.

Shine enhancers are oils used in spray form (often in an aerosol can). The can should be held

## Tips for applying hairspray:

| 1 | 2 | 3 | 4 | |
|---|---|---|---|---|
| Protect your eyes and face with your free hand while spraying. | Aim the spray so that the lacquer drops down on to the hair from above. | Spray the lacquer from a distance of 30cm (12in), so that a fine, even spray saturates the hair. | Spraying too close to the head will overdo one area, leaving blobs on the hair and sometimes causing it to droop with the weight. | **SAFETY TIP** Hair sprays are often flammable, so do not smoke when using them. Do not store them in direct heat or sunlight, and take care not to puncture the can. |

about 30cm (12in) away from the hair and sprayed above the head.

Waxes are used to give texture to the hair. Rub a small amount between the hands, allowing the friction to warm and melt the wax which should be quickly applied to the hair before it cools. It then becomes more solid, helping to hold the hair in position and give it a more textured look. Waxes are particularly useful on long hair with frizzy ends or on curly hair.

## HAIR-FIXING SPRAYS

Hair sprays commonly contain organic compounds that are synthesized to form plastic polymers (large molecules made up of simple but identical units). These polymers are dissolved in alcohol, which coat the hair with a clear plastic film.

Two of the polymers that are commonly used are polyvinyl pyrrolidone (PVP) and polyvinyl acetate (PVA). These are used in different ratios: 60 per cent PVP: 40 per cent PVA for normal use 70 per cent PVA: 30 per cent PVP for hard holding.

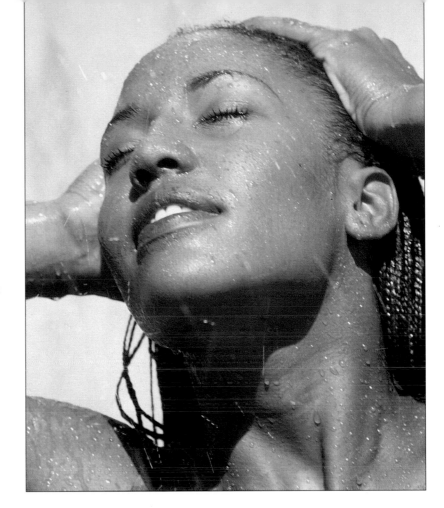

Examples of other polymer blends currently used in hair sprays are vinylacetate, crotonic acid, ethyl methacrylate and methacrylic acid. Since these polymers are acidic, a neutralizer is normally added, such as trisopropanolamine or 2-amino methyl propanol. The neutralizer also determines the strength or 'hold' of the hair spray. Hair sprays also contain perfumes and propellants, such as butane and propane.

When the lacquer is sprayed on to the hair, the alcohol evaporates and leaves the resin, or plastic coating, in the hair. This causes it to stick or glue together, thus holding the hair in place.

Always try to choose products packaged in aerosol cans that do not contain CFCs, the gases that destroy the ozone layer. Many manufacturers now also produce hand-pump hair sprays without propellant.

# Setting
# AND STYLING

**A**ll setting aids work by covering the hair shaft with a protective coating that when dry, helps to hold the shape that has been created and prevent the absorption of moisture into the air, thus making the hair keep its shape for longer.

Setting aids contain weak glues that hold the hair in place. Setting lotions are normally runny and can be difficult to apply, because they tend to drip everywhere. Gels contain chemicals that stiffen the product, but which become less viscous when rubbed on your hands. Mousses are foams that contain very small bubbles of air – the smaller the bubbles, the more dense the foam. They are often used for scrunch and natural drying.

Setting aids may use PVA and PVP in the same proportion as hair sprays, although natural gums are also used, such as tragacanth and karaya. Setting gels or mousses may frequently

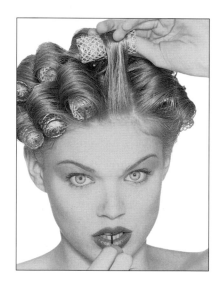

contain citric acid as a conditioner, hydrogenated castor oil, water (often referred to as 'aqua') and colour or perfume.

### STYLING TOOLS AND APPLIANCES
You can choose from a number of fashion appliances, tools and accessories. Some are basic items that everyone will need, such as combs and hairdriers; others – pins, clips, bands and rollers – are used for special styles of hair.

## PINS, CLIPS AND BANDS

These are indispensable for sectioning and securing hair during setting and cutting. Pins can also be used to hold hair in place while it is being styled. Double-pronged clips are usually used for making French pleats and other upswept styles.

Fine hair pins can easily be concealed in a finished style, but should only be used to secure a small amount of hair or the pins will slip and the hair escape. Most pins are available with untipped, plain ends or cushion-tipped ends, which are kinder on the scalp and less likely to break the hair. Most are made of metal or plastic.

Hair bands of various kinds can be used to secure the hair in ponytails, bunches and other more elaborate styles. These can be made of a variety of soft materials. Never use elastic rubber bands, as these can damage and split the hair.

## ROLLERS

Rollers are put into the hair after shampooing to curl it. Some are smooth, but those with spikes or brushes are the easiest to put in and secure. Some self-fix without the need for pins. The larger the roller, the more relaxed the curl of the hair.

Other kinds of shapers to curl the hair are made of soft plastic with wire inside, so that you can bend them into the required shape. They usually create a more natural look than rollers. Heated rollers can be used to curl the hair more readily. They should be used only on dry or very slightly damp hair.

Tongs consist of a barrel or prong, and a groove, into which the barrel fits. They can be used to create gentle waves or stronger curls in straight hair.

Straighteners consist of flat, heated plates to iron out frizz or curl, while crimpers have ridged metal plates that produce uniform patterned crimps in straight lines.

## STYLING AFRICAN CARIBBEAN HAIR

Many African Caribbean women dress their hair in traditional styles, such

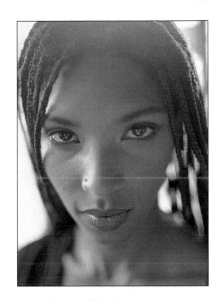

as cornrows or beading. The hair is twisted into dozens of tiny plaits or braids and, after the initial plaiting process, can be left for more than two months before it needs attention. Hair can also be threaded to create interesting effects. This involves twisting the hair and then threading a piece of cotton along it from the roots to the tips, before knotting it at the tip of the hair ends.

**SAFETY TIP**
Regular use of extremely hot tongs, crimpers and heated rollers can dry out and damage longer hair.

# Cutting and
# HOLIDAY HAIR CARE

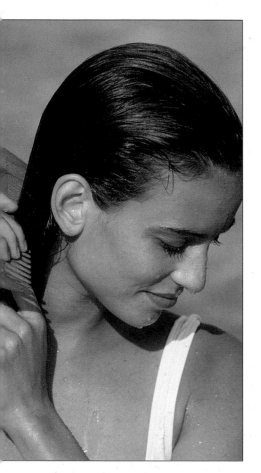

## CUTTING

Regular cutting of the hair is essential to keep it healthy. The ends of the hair tend to dry out, as they are furthest away from the scalp and are less protected by sebum. They are also the oldest part of the hair shaft, so they have suffered from more weathering. Chemicals and pollutants in the environment, the sun, chlorine, and the effects of brushing also tend to damage the ends of the hair, so regular trimming is essential to keep your hair looking healthy.

It is a good idea to have your hair cut before you go on holiday, or, if not, as soon as you come back.

## HOLIDAY HAIR CARE

Two weeks in the sun, with plenty of swimming in a pool or the sea, can cause more damage to the hair than is done in the whole of the rest of the year.

The ultraviolet rays of the sun damage the cuticle and deplete the natural oils and moisture in the hair. Strong winds whip up hair, causing it to tangle, break and split at the ends. Chlorinated and salt water also damage the hair, especially when the hair is not shampooed or rinsed immediately after bathing.

Protecting your hair against the sun is almost as important as protecting your skin, so wear a sun-hat or headscarf on the beach. If you want your locks to be free, you can buy protective hair sprays or sun-screen gels that contain

### CUTTING: HOW OFTEN ?

Even if you are growing your hair long, the ends should be trimmed regularly – every six weeks or at least every two months – to keep it in the best possible condition and make it easier to look after.

a UVB screen (ultraviolet B being the most intense and damaging form of ultraviolet light). Remember to reapply sprays or gels after swimming. Or you can use a leave-in conditioner that protects the hair against UVBs

On windy days, keep your hair tied back or up to prevent tangles. Long hair can be plaited or braided and left like this all day. Remember to wear a sun-hat or screen when shopping or sightseeing, as well as when you are on the beach.

When your hair has been in the sunshine all day, try to leave it to dry naturally after washing and shampooing it. It is best to wash your hair frequently, especially after bathing, so remember to use a frequent-wash shampoo. If you are bathing in a swimming pool, use an anti-chlorine shampoo.

## WINTER HOLIDAYS
Winter holidays can be harmful for your hair, too. Sunshine on the ski-slopes is often stronger than the midday summer sun. Harsh, biting winds can cause

damage, while central heating tends to make the air drier and causes the hair to lose moisture. Extreme cold makes the hair brittle and dry. To reduce the damage done by central heating, place humidifiers on radiators at home to increase the water

vapour in the air; when you are away, place a bowl of water by the radiator and replenish it frequently. Use a more intensive conditioner in winter to combat the dryness caused by cold. On the ski-slopes, use a UVB screen on your hair, or wear a hat.

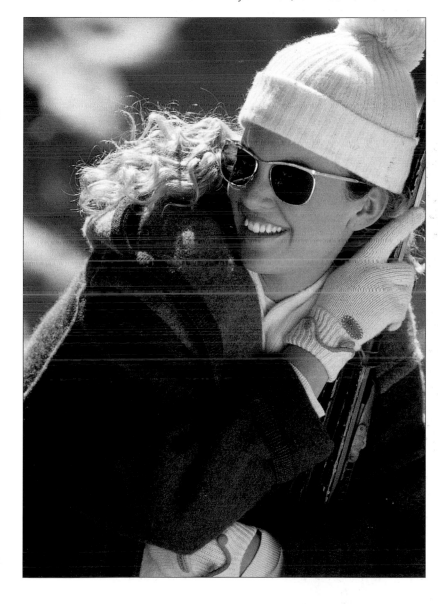

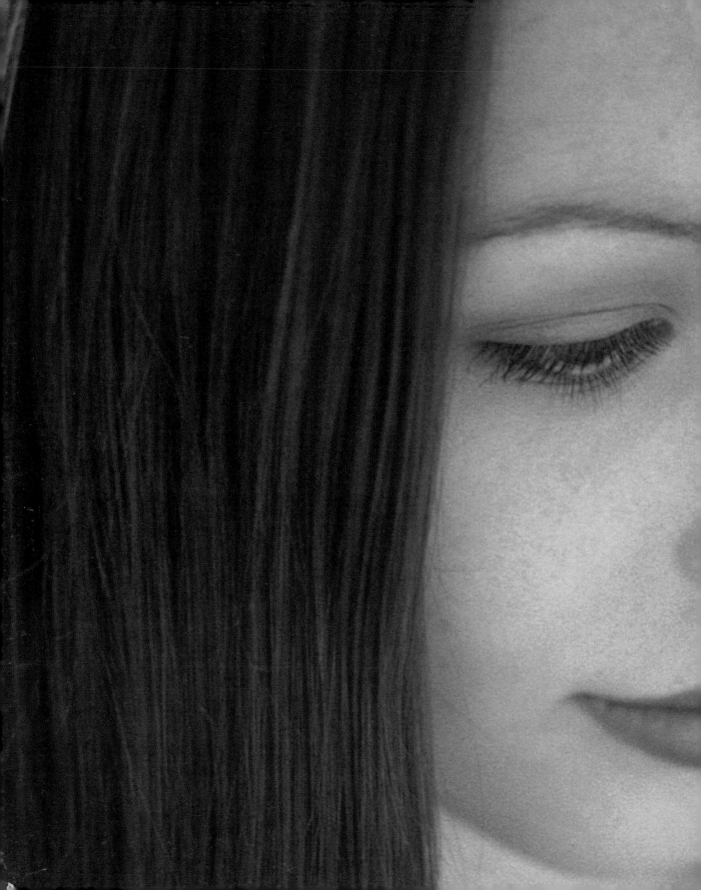

# HAIR
# Health

# Health
# FROM THE INSIDE

Beautiful hair needs to be nourished from within. The truism that we are what we eat is certainly relevant for our hair. Healthy hair depends on our general well-being and on a well-balanced diet containing sufficient protein, iron and other minerals and vitamins. Regular exercise is also important as it promotes good circulation of blood to the scalp, ensuring that vital oxygen and nutrients get to the follicles and the roots of the hair.

## VITAL PROTEIN AND IRON

An adequate amount of protein in the diet is essential for healthy hair. Good sources of protein include lean meat, poultry, fish, cheese, eggs and milk, as well as nuts, seeds and pulses. Red meat is the best source of iron as well as protein, although vegetarians can get iron from pulses; green vegetables such as spinach, beans and broccoli; and nuts, seeds and dried fruit like apricots. Vegetarians need to eat plenty of dairy products and soya to keep their protein levels up.

There is some evidence that people who originally ate meat but have since become vegetarian are less able to extract all the iron they need from vegetable sources alone.

Iron is one of the most necessary minerals for healthy hair, and yet many women are low on iron stores. Monthly menstruation means that women should constantly replenish their iron, otherwise levels of this vital mineral will fall. One recent study showed that as many as 80–90 per cent of women of childbearing age who suffer from hair loss are at least mildly anaemic. Women in this age group should make sure that they eat a wide range of iron-rich food. It is also a good idea for women to have their blood iron levels checked from time to time, especially during pregnancy, after childbirth, and if they have frequent or heavy periods.

Tea and coffee hamper the absorption of iron from the gut. If you are taking iron supplements, it's particularly important that you do not drink tea or coffee at the same time, or within half an hour of taking your iron tablet. Vitamin C, on the other hand, helps the absorption of iron, so it is a good idea to make sure that you get enough vitamin C or take supplements alongside your iron.

Alcohol may also hamper the absorption of vitamins and minerals that are crucial for healthy hair. It is known that alcohol raises the level of male hormones in the body, but there is no clinical evidence that this is connected with the development of hair loss in some women. Some contraceptive pills also deplete the B-complex vitamins and zinc, which are both important for the health of the hair.

## OTHER ESSENTIAL NUTRIENTS

Fruit is packed with minerals and vitamins, so try to eat at least three pieces of fruit each day, together with a couple of portions of vegetables. If you need a snack, try nuts and grains or seeds – sometimes found in mucoli-type bars – instead of biscuits.

While dairy foods are high in protein, they also contain a lot of fat, especially the saturated fats that are less good for health. You may like to cut down on saturated fats, but it is a myth that a diet high in fat will cause an overproduction of sebum, leading to lank, greasy or oily hair. Choose low-fat yoghurts or semi-skimmed milk, rather than the full-fat varieties, but don't overdo it – it's important

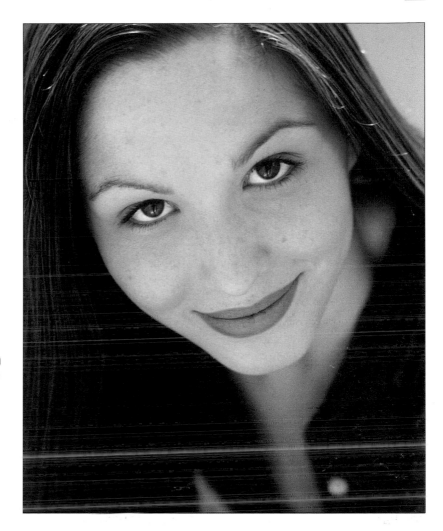

to remember that you do need some fat in the diet to absorb the fat-soluble vitamins A, D and E.

Amino acids, the building blocks of protein, are essential in our diet and necessary for healthy hair growth. Some are known as 'essential amino acids', because they cannot be made in the body but must

be included in the diet. First-class protein, such as that found in meat, dairy products, eggs and fish, contains significant quantities of all the amino acids. Second-class protein, such as that found in vegetables, pulses and seeds, contains only some of the essential amino acids, which is why a vegetarian diet must include a wide range of foods.

# DEFICIENCIES and remedies

## NUTRITION

Nutritional deficiencies sufficient to cause hair problems in the Western world are few; but there are some worth mentioning.

## IRON

The most common deficiency is of iron, and when it does become serious, hair loss may occur. Women of childbearing age are prone to develop iron deficiency anaemia because of the need to replace the iron lost every month through menstruation.

## ZINC

Zinc deficiency may also cause hair loss and a scaling scalp, but this is more likely to be due to malabsorption than to a deficiency of intake. In clinical observations, extreme zinc deficiency causes hair loss; it can also cause problems with the skin in the nasolabial areas (the folds on either side of the nose) and around the mouth, with inflammation and soreness. And in very extreme circumstances (rarely seen in the West) scaly scalps may a problem. Although these effects are extremely unlikely to occur, you should make sure that you get enough zinc in your diet, or take supplements.

## COPPER

Copper deficiency is extremely rare in the Western world, although it can cause a rare hair problem known as Menkes' kinky hair syndrome.

## VITAMIN B12

Lack of vitamin B12 inhibits iron absorption and is therefore implicated in hair loss. Pernicious anaemia is a condition where the stomach lining is defective and cannot absorb vitamin B12 properly, thereby causing hair loss. The condition can be successfully treated with supplements of a special form of vitamin B12 called hydroxocobalamin.

Overconsumption of some vitamins may equally cause problems, since they accumulate in the body and you can actually overdose on them. Vitamin A is the most common culprit, and an overdose can result when people have taken too many supplements, sometimes resulting in hair loss.

## ESSENTIAL FATTY ACIDS

Essential fatty acids, linoleic and alpha-linoleic acid are vital for health and cannot be made by the body, so they need to be included in your diet. Linoleic acid is found in a wide range of foodstuffs, especially vegetables and grains; alpha-linoleic acid is found in wheat, beans and spinach. Eicosapentanoeic acid and docosahexanoic acid are also essential fatty acids, which are primarily found in seafood and safflower oil. If you are in doubt about whether you're getting enough, you can take supplements, such as fish oil and evening primrose oil.

### SAFETY TIP

Excessive amounts of vitamin A, taken as a supplement, can actually cause hair loss.

!

# where to find the
# VITAMINS AND MINERALS YOU NEED

| | TYPE | LOCATION |
|---|---|---|
| 1 | Zinc | Oysters, ginger root, red meat, pecans, split peas, brazil nuts, egg yolks, wholewheat and rye. You can also take zinc supplements. |
| 2 | Iron | Red meat, liver, spinach, egg yolks, pulses, cocoa, cane molasses, shellfish and parsley. Iron supplements may also be taken. Many women, especially those with heavy periods or pregnant women, are anaemic. Drinking tea and coffee hampers the absorption of iron, but vitamin C boosts its intake (see below). |
| 3 | Vitamin C | Vitamin C assists in the absorption of essential minerals such as iron and zinc. It is found in most fruit, and especially in citrus and some exotic fruit, in rosehips, green vegetables such as broccoli, Brussels sprouts and cauliflower, liver, kidney and potatoes. Foods should not be stored for long and should be lightly cooked, as this vitamin is water-soluble. Vitamin C supplements are readily available. |
| 4 | Vitamin B12 | Liver, meat, fish, dairy produce and eggs. It is also present in brewer's yeast, or you can take supplements. |
| 5 | Vitamin A | This vitamin helps to keep the scalp healthy. It is found in apricots, peaches, spinach, liver, beef and lamb. |
| 6 | Vitamin E | This vitamin serves as an antioxidant for vitamin A – that is, it prevents vitamin A from oxidizing, or decomposing. Vitamin E is found in butter, wholemeal cereals, broccoli and margarine (from corn oil). |
| 7 | Biotin | The condition known as seborrhoeic dermatitis (see p.69) has been linked to a low intake of biotin. It is found in liver, kidney, egg yolks, yeast and yeast extracts, pulses and nuts. |

# THE EFFECTS of dieting, stress and ageing

Many modern women diet almost constantly in an attempt to achieve the kind of figure that is promoted in beauty, health and fitness magazines.

## THE DANGERS OF DIETING

Young women often try one diet after another, using many of the crash diets that are in vogue – the low-carbohydrate diet, the high-fibre diet, the high-protein diet, and so on. Others rely on special slimming foods and meals with reduced calories. Many women intend to diet, but then become so hungry that they break the programme – often with an unhealthy snack which gives them the sugar boost they may crave. Then, feeling guilty at having broken their diet, they begin again with renewed strictness the next day.

Such dieting can be very unhealthy. It is far better, when trying to achieve a firm body that is not overweight, to take regular exercise and eat well-balanced meals. Even if you supplement with vitamin pills while dieting, these vitamins and minerals are often not absorbed as well as they are in a healthy diet. If you are cutting right down on fats, for instance, your body will not absorb the fat-soluble vitamins. A balanced diet with a little fat and a low sugar intake is without doubt the best diet for the body and hair.

## STRESS AND POLLUTION FACTORS

Today's hectic lifestyles and the focus on staying slim have taken a heavy toll on women's health. Stress is a factor in many modern illnesses and is known to be linked to hair growth. Stress hormones can affect the growth of hair and can even lead to dramatic hair loss. An increasing number of young women in their 20s and 30s are experiencing premature thinning, or loss of hair. In other women, stress leads to a poor diet, which means that women do not eat enough protein, minerals and vitamins, and end up with dry, lack-lustre and brittle hair. Crash dieting can lead to

quite dramatic hair loss three months later. Because of the growth cycle of the hair, it takes that long before the effect of any major stress is actually seen on the hair. As a result, people often do not make a direct link between the hair loss and the cause. Anorexia and other eating disorders often also lead to hair loss.

The modern world is not always friendly to our hair, either. Many of the chemicals and pollutants in the environment can cling to it and damage it, especially if not washed out quickly. Cigarette smoke in particular can adhere to the hair and stain it yellow. Alcohol and other drugs can affect the absorption of vitamins and minerals and therefore reduce hair growth.

## THE AGEING GAME

Unfortunately, as we grow older our hair changes – usually not for the better. The main effects of ageing are that the hair becomes thinner and (usually from the age of

35 onwards) white hairs start to appear. Women frequently start to tint or perm the hair as they become older and this may cause damage if it is carried out excessively, because the hair becomes dry and brittle.

It is very important that as you age, you take greater care of your hair, your skin and your health. Young women may be able to get away with eating poorly, exercising erratically, and smoking and drinking, because their bodies have greater powers of recuperation. With age, however, your body becomes less resilient and you need to look after yourself much more carefully.

There is nothing you can do to prevent your hair from greying, as this is genetically determined. However, most women can retain their youthful looks by means of highlighting and tinting (see pp.98–101) to conceal the effects of white hairs.

Women's hair usually becomes thinner between the ages of 30 and 50, but increased hair loss in your 40s, 50s and 60s may be a sign of a mineral or vitamin deficiency or of poor general health. If you suffer from hair loss at this age, see your doctor or a reputable trichologist.

Sometimes hormone replacement therapy can affect the hair (see p.59), and if this is the case then you should consult your doctor and perhaps change to another type.

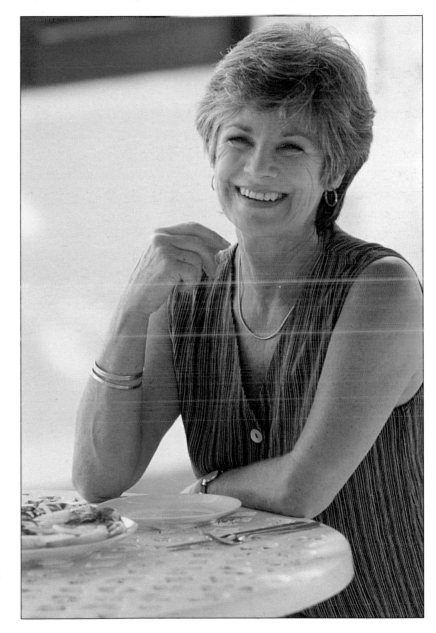

# All about
# TRICHOLOGISTS

If you have a serious problem with your hair or scalp, you may be referred to, or decide to visit a trichologist.

Unfortunately this profession is not regulated in the UK, which means that anyone can set up in business and call themselves a trichologist. Some of these people may be unscrupulous and may recommend expensive and ineffective treatments for a wide range of problems, from premature balding to dandruff. However, the Institute of Trichologists in London is currently seeking state registration and has already made an application to the government for this.

It is important that you check that any British trichologist whom you consult is a member of the Institute of Trichologists. The Institute regulates its members through training, in the first instance, and through a strict Code of Ethics. This means that they will have undertaken a course of study – normally three years – and will have passed the institute's rigorous examinations. All members are then registered with the institute and must abide by its Code of Ethics. Watch out for those who would fool you. If you are asked to pay for a course of treatments in advance, beware! It is against the Code of Ethics to do this, and such trichologists are probably not members of the institute. If in doubt, give the institute a call – it will be happy to send you a list of registered members.

Since the US has no equivalent organization to the Institute of Trichologists, most American trichologists are trained either in the UK or through courses run by the International Association of Trichologists, which originated in the US but is now based in Australia. However, they may not be allowed to carry out treatments in the US unless they have also trained as cosmetologists.

Trichologists can help with a range of hair problems, from those caused by excessive perming and tinting to hair loss caused by a wide variety of causes. They will also know when you should be referred to a doctor, dermatologist or other medical specialist. Your general practitioner may not be particularly interested in a hair-loss problem (perhaps because this is often deemed cosmetic) and will usually be able to see you for only a short time anyway. When you visit a trichologist, he or she

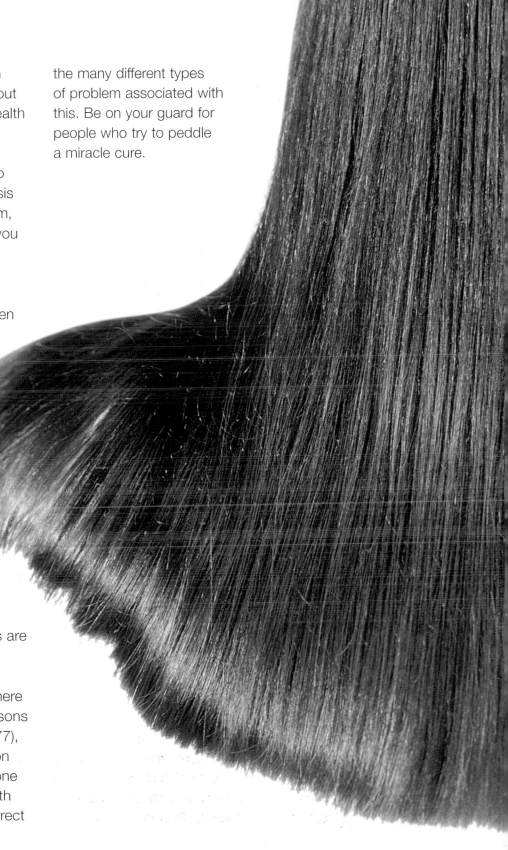

will spend as much as an hour with you, talking about everything from diet to health and medication, and examining your hair and scalp. Trichologists aim to achieve a correct diagnosis for your particular problem, and this may mean that you need to have blood tests carried out.

Once a diagnosis has been made, it may be that the trichologist is able to deal with it, or that you need medical assistance, in which case you may be referred back to your doctor or to a dermatologist. Some of the Institute of Trichologists' members are also doctors of medicine, in which case such referrals are not necessary.

It should be noted that there are a vast number of reasons for hair loss (see pp.58–77), to name just one common hair problem. Therefore one treatment sold to deal with hair loss is unlikely to correct

the many different types of problem associated with this. Be on your guard for people who try to peddle a miracle cure.

# Hair problems:

# ALOPECIA

The term 'alopecia' simply means hair loss. It is used to cover any form of hair loss, whatever the cause.

### ANDROGENIC ALOPECIA (MALE-PATTERN BALDNESS)

While always common in men, this condition was not seen so often in women until recently, although now it seems to be on the increase. It can occur as the result of hormonal changes, but appears to be getting more prevalent due to the stressful, hectic lifestyles that women lead today. A tendency to hair loss of this type seems to be

inherited in women, just as it is in men. In women the condition normally creates extensive hair thinning, rather than actual baldness, though the latter does occasionally occur.

If androgenic hair loss occurs after the menopause, the cause is usually genetic. In younger women, however, research has linked this type of hair loss to stress. Too much stress causes a rise in adrenalin and in the male hormones known as androgens, such as testosterone. Alcohol also

raises testosterone levels, so women who drink a lot may also be more liable to suffer from hair loss, although there is no evidence to prove this.

Hair loss in women usually starts at the front of the hair, on the temples, then moves across the top of the head and down the sides, although the hair usually remains thick at the nape of the neck; in men the hair loss does not affect the sides of the head, but begins on the frontal hairline and then affects the crown, and from there the two areas ultimately join.

## DIFFERENT TYPES OF ALOPECIA

**'PATTERN' BALDNESS**
This is most common in men and affects about 40 per cent of men by the age of 40; in women it takes a slightly different form.

*1*

**ALOPECIA AREATA**
Where patches of hair fall out, for poorly understood reasons, although it is known to be an auto-immune disorder.

*2*

**TRACTION ALOPECIA**
Where hair is pulled out at the roots by hairstyles that constantly drag it back tightly, or by nervous twisting of the hair.

*3*

**ALOPECIA FROM SCARRING**
Where the skin is damaged on the scalp and forms a scar on which no hair will grow.

*4*

There are a vast number of other reasons for hair loss, ranging from poor diet and the use of certain medications to post-operative and post-partum problems.

*5*

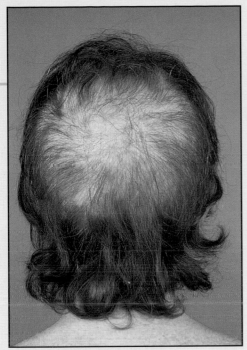

*Alopecia can be unsightly and may cause a great deal of distress to the sufferer.*

## POST-MENOPAUSAL THINNING

After the menopause women's hair can begin to thin, because their levels of the female hormone oestrogen fall in proportion to the level of androgens in the bloodstream. Hormone replacement therapy (HRT) can improve this condition, but it does depend on the type of the hormones used. Oestrogen-only HRT is now recommended solely for women who have had their womb removed; most other forms of HRT involve taking a progestogen (one of a group of steroid hormones used in oral contraceptives). Some of these (such as cyproterone acetate and medroxy-progesterone acetate) are less likely to cause hair loss, while others (such as norethisterone and levonorgestrel) are more masculine in their effect.

These synthetic progestogens tend to be broken down by the body into testosterone, so they can have virilizing effects, such as thinning the hair and increasing facial hair. Women who experience these problems with HRT can take natural progesterone instead, either through skin patches or through creams or gels, which can be rubbed on to the skin or inserted into the vagina.

## CONTRACEPTIVE PILLS

The contraceptive pill is also sometimes linked to hair loss – again, this may depend on the type of progestogen used. If a woman experiences hair loss while she is on the pill, she should switch to a brand that contains one of the more hair-friendly progestogens. If that doesn't help, she could consider an alternative form of contraception.

## HORMONAL DISORDERS

Some illnesses cause an overproduction of hormones, which in turn may lead to thinning hair. One such illness is polycystic ovaries; there are at least six causes for this disorder, which strangely does not always involve the existence of a cyst.

Treatment of the condition depends on the dominant symptom – among many other symptoms, there is an increase in a hormone called androstenedione and also in oestradiol and testosterone, which can result in facial hair, acne and the loss of scalp hair.

Other illnesses that can affect hair growth, and occasionally cause excessive growth of hair on the face and body, are disorders of the pituitary gland.

# ALOPECIA areata

Alopecia areata results in the appearance of roughly circular bald patches on the scalp. The skin in the affected area is smooth and soft and has no hair at all. There is no disturbance of the skin (as in the case of skin disorders, which may also cause temporary hair loss). Itching frequently precedes the hair loss, and the patches not only affect the scalp hair, but eyebrows, eyelashes and body hair can also be lost. Bald patches may appear on the arms and legs and, in men, beard hair may be lost.

## AN AUTO-IMMUNE DISORDER

The condition is a bit of a mystery – just why it happens is not fully understood, although it can be caused by a sudden shock (which very rarely may cause dramatic total hair loss). Alopecia areata can sometimes be linked to a thyroid malfunction or to an untreated abscess on the tooth. It is now known to be an auto-immune disorder,

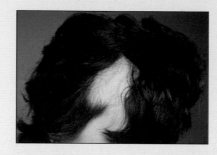

*A typical bald patch caused by alopecia areata.*

and there is commonly a hereditary factor. Research has shown that in alopecia areata the hair follicles in the anagen growing phase become a target for attack by auto-immune cells. Hair loss is sudden: sometimes even overnight. The healthy hairs break off just above the surface of the scalp, leaving hairs that look like little exclamation marks when viewed under a microscope. Then these hairs fall out. There is no loss of the hair follicles themselves; these simply fail to produce hair, either temporarily or, if the condition is prolonged, permanently.

Alopecia areata may be no more than a few bald patches

that appear and then regrow hair. If the patches are small, the chances of regrowth are very good. Sometimes it affects only the pigmented hair, so that white hairs remain.

Since severe shock may cause dramatic hair loss, this may explain someone's hair going white overnight – all the pigmented hairs are lost, but not the white ones. Often, when the hair grows back after alopecia areata, they are white to begin with, but pigmented hairs then commonly replace them.

Diffuse alopecia areata leads to sudden thinning without the bald patches. This condition is far less common than the bald patches described above. 'Alopecia totalis' is the term used when all the hair on the head is affected, and 'alopecia universalis' when all the body hair is affected, too. When this happens, the chances of regrowth are poor.

## ALLEVIATING THE PROBLEM

There is no foolproof treatment for alopecia areata, because the cause is so poorly understood. Stress seems to perpetuate the condition, so anything that alleviates stress is beneficial.

Changing your lifestyle or having stress-relieving treatments such as massage, aromatherapy and other complementary treatments can be successful. A great help is simply getting a correct diagnosis and explanation – an hour's session with a trichologist can be extremely reassuring.

Those treatments that do exist are aimed at producing new growth, as prevention of the disorder is not yet possible, and there are some remedies that may make a difference. Some scalp stimulants can have an effect: methyl nicotinate or minoxidil (sold as 'Regaine') may help. Sometimes steroid creams are prescribed and some dermatologists will try steroid injections into the bald patches. These treatments may help in some cases, but not in others.

There are also a number of more natural remedies that have recently been used to treat alopecia areata. These are not well researched, but if they are harmless they may be worth a try.

Alopecia areata is not harmful, but it can be extremely distressing. Women may change their whole lifestyles because they are ashamed to reveal their thin, patchy or absent hair and a few may even become suicidal. If you experience this kind of hair loss, seek advice from a reputable trichologist (see pp.56–7).

## TRACTION ALOPECIA

Traction alopecia usually occurs in women who wear severe hairstyles where the hair is pulled back tightly into a bun, pleat or ponytail. It can also occur in black women who wear their hair in cornrows or beads. These problems happen only when the traction is prolonged, in which case the hair is pulled out at the roots, especially along the front hairline, at partings and at the sides of the head. A new hairstyle will usually resolve the problem,

although if the traction has gone on for a long time, then the hair loss may be permanent.

In other cases a woman develops a nervous habit of pulling, tugging or winding the hair, which draws the hairs out by the roots. Some people deliberately pull out individual hairs – this is like other nervous habits, such as biting the fingernails, and is usually repeated subconsciously. Stress-relieving treatments and hypnosis can be very useful in dealing with this problem.

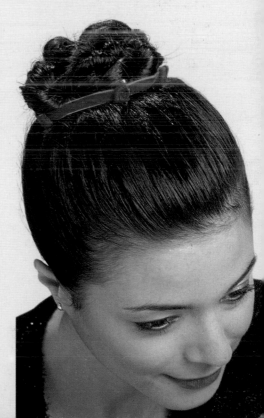

# Hair loss

## TREATMENTS

First and foremost, get a good diagnosis. Where there is a hormonal problem in women, treatment will generally arrest the hair loss.

### ANDROGENIC ALOPECIA

The treatment for men and women is very different. For men there is only cosmetic treatment, as to date the cause cannot be treated.

Women, on the other hand, can have hormonal treatment, which may regrow hair or at least arrest its loss. Common to both sexes is the drug minoxidil, which has to be used repeatedly.

### Topical minoxidil

This drug was developed to treat high blood pressure, but it was found that a side-effect was increased hair growth. It is sold as 'Regaine' and is the most commonly used drug for male- and female-pattern baldness. At least four months' treatment is required before any effects are seen; new growth may be soft and downy at first, and may remain that way, never forming normal terminal hairs. The treatment has to be continued for the effect to last – as soon as it is stopped, the hair will be lost again.

### Retin-A/tretinoin

Tretinoin is sold as retin-A for the treatment of acne and other skin disorders. Studies have shown that retin-A combined with minoxidil can result in moderate hair regrowth in cases of both pattern baldness and alopecia areata.

### HAIR TRANSPLANTS
### (not suitable for Alopecia Areata sufferers)

Hair-transplant surgery, when carried out by an expert, can redistribute hair very well. Narrow strips of scalp, including the hair follicles, are taken from areas where there is dense hair (usually at the back of the head) and moved to areas where the hair is thin or non-existent. They are replaced after sectioning, either in groups of four or five hairs or one at a time. There is even pioneering work being done on transplanting into scar tissue, which is brilliant treatment for a scarred scalp or beard. However, always make sure that the surgeon is medically qualified, as there are some charlatans practising in this area.

## Cyproterone acetate with ethinyloestradiol

This can be used as a hormonal contraceptive pill. In its normally prescribed form it can also be used to treat acne and excessive facial hair, plus androgenic alopecia in women. Higher doses than are normally prescribed for acne are now used to treat this condition and there is a good success rate in those patients who are suitable for the treatment.

## ALOPECIA AREATA

A range of different treatments is available to attempt to alleviate this complex problem.

## Corticosteroids

This is the most common form of treatment for alopecia areata today. In mild cases corticosteroid creams are used, which are applied to the area of hair loss. An alternative is injections of steroids into the scalp, just below the skin close to the hair follicle. These injections are repeated approximately once a month, and it may take up to two months before any new hair growth is noticed. Systemic corticosteroids can be used where hair loss is dramatic and sudden and may be given as tablets or by injection every four to six weeks. Cortisone taken internally is a powerful drug and can have adverse side-effects; it needs careful monitoring.

## Puva

This treatment involves taking a psoralen (usually Methoxsalen) – a light-sensitive drug – and undergoing short exposure to UVA or long-wave ultraviolet light. The success rate has been estimated to be as high as 40–60 per cent, with the response being best when hair loss is recent. Treatment normally lasts for between three and six months, with two to three five-minute treatments a week.

## Immunosuppressive drugs

Because alopecia areata is an auto-immune disorder, treatment with immuno-suppressive drugs, such as cyclosporin, has been attempted. However, the main problem is that it leaves the patient vulnerable to infections and tumours, so its use is not generally recommended.

## Irritants

When irritants are applied to the scalp, the reaction draws the T-lymphocytes (white blood cells, which in alopecia areata turn rogue and attack the cells of the hair follicles) away from the follicles, which may then regrow new hair. Research is being done to see whether this could be developed as a treatment for alopecia areata.

## Retin-A/tretinoin and topical minoxidil

These products have also been used to treat alopecia areata.

## Zinc

Zinc seems to have an effect on the immune system and may help in some cases of alopecia areata. It is also used in disorders related to the male hormone dihydrotestosterone and may be useful in treating male and female pattern baldness. The topical application of zinc may also reduce sebum production.

# MIRACLE CURES for hair loss

These are some of the remedies that are sold to reverse hair loss. However, there is no medical evidence that any of them work, so they may be a waste of time and money.

### GREEN TEA

Green tea contains powerful antioxidants called polyphenols, which scavenge free radicals. It also contains carotenoids and may inhibit the action of male hormones in the body.

### NIZORAL/KETOCONAZOLE

This is used to treat fungal infections of the skin. Nizoral shampoo contains ketoconazole, and is used in the treatment of severe dandruff and fungal infections of the scalp, for which it works well. There is no evidence that it affects hair loss in women.

### SKINORAN/AZELAIC ACID

This is used to treat acne and related conditions, for which it is effective. Because of its anti-androgenic effects, its use in the treatment of pattern baldness is being researched, but there is no evidence that it has any efficacy.

### TAGAMET/CIMETIDINE

Cimetidine is sold under the brand-name Tagamet to treat stomach ulcers and related conditions. It has been suggested that it may cause hair growth, but there is no scientific proof of this.

### SAW PALMETTO OIL

This comes from the berries of a species of palm tree, and studies have shown the oil to act as a potent anti-androgen. Products are now being sold containing saw palmetto oil for the treatment of pattern baldness. There is no evidence that they work.

### GAMMA LINOLEIC ACID

Gamma linoleic acid plays an important part in regulating androgen action in target cells, and it has been suggested that it is used to treat disorders related to the male hormone dihydro-testosterone, such as acne, pattern baldness and excessive facial hair. There is no evidence that it is effective, although it is harmless and may be useful as a general supplement.

### POLYSORBATE 80

This is used as a cleanser in many commercial hair products and can cause the release of histamines, which it has been suggested may be involved in promoting hair growth. There is no proof that it works.

### EMU OIL

This contains a high level of linoleic acid, which research has shown to be an effective anti-androgen. It has also been shown to increase pigmentation in the hair of some animals. Hair restoration products containing emu oil have recently been patented. Again, there is no scientific proof of their effectiveness.

### VITAMIN B6

Vitamin B6 may be of some help to people who suffer from some types of hair loss.

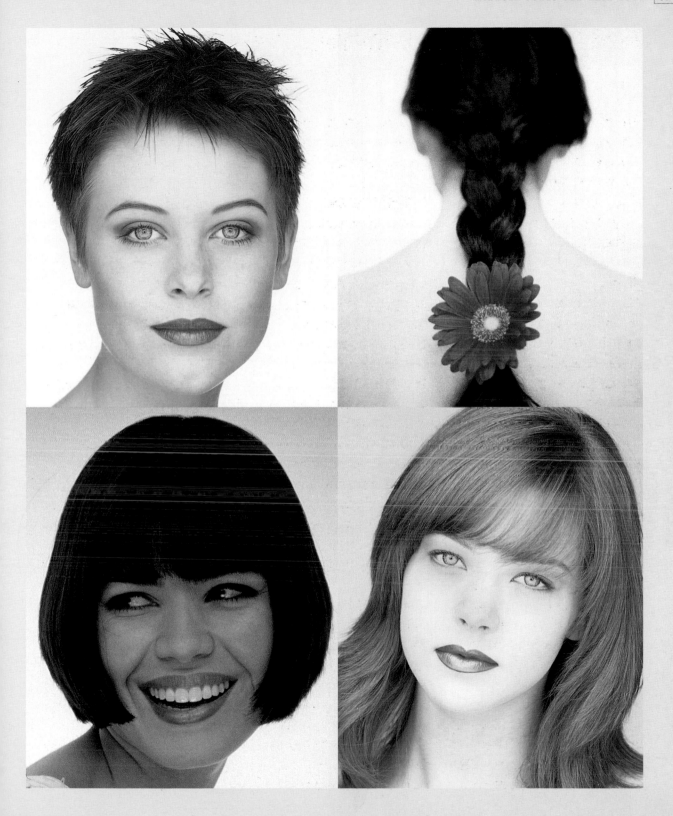

# HAIR LOSS from cancer treatment

It is well known that sudden and dramatic hair loss occurs as a result of radiotherapy and chemotherapy treatment for cancer.

## THE EFFECTS OF CHEMOTHERAPY

Chemotherapy is used to destroy the fast-growing cancer cells, but it also tends to affect other fast-growing cells in the body, such as those that produce the hair (causing hair loss) and those in the gut (producing diarrhoea, nausea and vomiting). Because chemotherapy attacks the rapidly dividing cells, 90 per cent of actively growing hairs tend to be shed, leaving the remaining 10 per cent in the resting phase. Some hair follicles do not shed the hair, but produce narrower, weaker strands that break off easily.

This hair loss is only a temporary condition and the hair will grow back to normal when the treatment is over. In fact, many people say that their hair grows back thicker and healthier than it was before. Sometimes the hair is of a different texture, being straighter or curlier than the original hair; sometimes it may even be a different colour. These apparent changes may, however, be due to the fact that we tend to judge hair on its appearance when it is longer, has been faded by the sun or straightened with its own weight, so that these differences do not always last. Hair is often curlier when very short. It is also possible that the chemotherapy drugs have interfered with the development of the cells at the base of the hair.

Hair loss caused by chemotherapy is usually sudden. It may happen overnight, with the patient waking up to find large clumps of hair on their pillow. Because of this, many people who expect to experience hair loss have their hair cut very short, to minimize the amount lost and so that their appearance doesn't change so dramatically. Some patients even choose to shave their head, since they prefer a completely bald head to a patchy-looking scalp.

With some cancers, a cold cap can be used on the scalp to reduce circulation to the head. This prevents the toxic chemicals in the blood from reaching the hair follicles. The cold cap is frozen and applied to the hair, then left on for as long as possible (up to two hours), depending on the chemicals used and the time it takes for the body to eliminate most of them.

The cap will need replacing after one hour to keep the scalp cold enough. Sometimes it is advised that the hair is wetted before application of the cap. While this treatment is extremely uncomfortable, it can help reduce or prevent hair loss, so most women want to give it a try. However, in some cancers, such as leukaemia, the chemicals must be allowed to circulate to all parts of the body and hair loss is inevitable.

## CHEMOTHERAPY DRUGS MOST LIKELY TO CAUSE HAIR LOSS

Amsacrine, Cytosine arabinoside, Cyclophosphamide, Doxorubicin, Epirubicin, Etoposide, Paclitaxel (Taxol), used in ovarian and breast cancer; Ifosfamide, Vincristine, Bleomycins. (These often cause hair loss, though not always.)

## CHEMOTHERAPY DRUGS LESS LIKELY TO CAUSE HAIR LOSS

Actinomycin, Cisplatin, Daunorubicin, Methotrexate, Carboplatin, Mitomycine C, Vinblastine.

## WIGS

Many women choose to wear a wig while they are bald, at least when they are outside the house; others wear a headscarf or hat. Some women prefer to start wearing a wig before they lose their hair and continue to do so until their hair has grown back to a reasonable length; others enjoy the novelty of an ultra-short hairstyle. There is a wide range of wigs available, ranging from those made with natural hair to synthetic ones of varying degrees of quality.

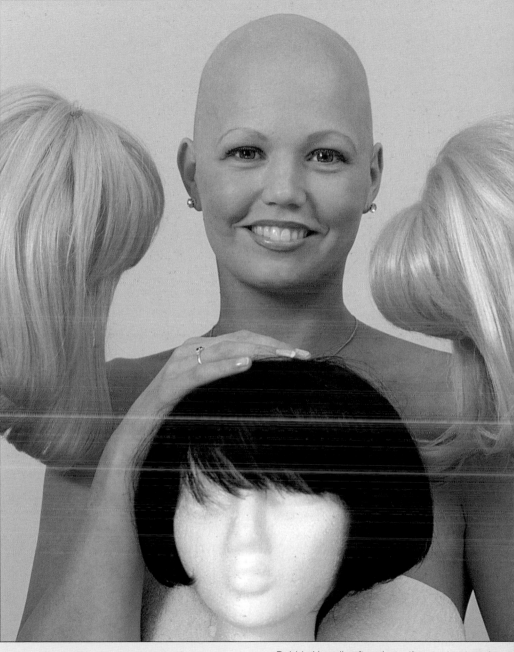

*Debbie Howells after chemotherapy treatment.*

# Disorders
# OF THE SCALP

There are a number of skin conditions that have repercussions on the way the scalp looks.

### PSORIASIS

This is a skin condition that varies from mild to severe and even disfiguring. It is a genetically inherited disorder, and is the result of a reduction or total absence of one layer of the epidermis

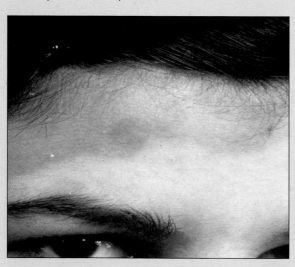

*Seborrhoeic eczema forms a mass of greasy scales and can be unsightly.*

(the outer layer of the skin). The symptoms are patches of thickened, silver-coloured scales, with the skin appearing red underneath. There is usually no hair loss, unless the condition is very severe, but psoriasis on the scalp can be distressing. It may cause itching and scratching, and this in turn can lead to the loss of some hair. There may also be temporary hair loss if the scalp becomes infected. Treatment is normally with a coal-tar product or dithrenol BP, which should be left on the hair for some time. In more severe cases ultraviolet light is used.

### ECZEMA

This is a common skin condition that results in red, itchy patches on the skin and sometimes on the scalp. It varies from mild cases, where the skin is sensitive and dry, easily irritated and forms a rash, to severe cases, with red, scaly, raw, weeping and even bleeding patches.

The most common kind of eczema is known as 'atopic', meaning that the individual is born with the condition, as opposed to developing it later in life or as the result of a specific allergy.

Eczema is most common in children. It is basically an allergic condition and the tendency to develop eczema usually runs in families. The condition is becoming more common, and this may be due to an increase in artificial chemicals in the air and in foodstuffs. Recently it has been suggested that the increase may be linked to the fact that children are becoming more and more protected from germs, so that their immune systems tend to become active against substances that are normally harmless. Eczema is often triggered by food allergies (dairy products being the most common trigger).

If you suffer from eczema, it is important to keep the skin moist by using aqueous creams on the skin and specially prepared bath oils. Steroid creams are normally prescribed for severe cases.

If eczema is severe, the skin can be broken and is liable to infection with bacteria, in which case it needs treatment with antibiotics. It can also become infected with the cold-sore virus, leading to a dangerous illness called eczema herpeticum.

There is also a form of eczema that is called 'seborrhoeic eczema' (also known as 'cradle cap' in babies). This forms a dense mass of brown, greasy scales on top of the head. It usually disappears by the age of two. It is common in adults and may be caused by an allergy to sebum, but it is also connected to hormones. It is recommended that sufferers wash their hair every day with an extremely mild shampoo.

Alcohol and spicy foods often exacerbate the seborrhoeic condition. It is sometimes necessary to eat very small quantities of the substance concerned, since otherwise you can suffer a massive allergic response if you accidentally eat something containing it.

## CONTACT ECZEMA OR DERMATITIS

This condition is peculiar to the individual, in that it is a reaction to a product that is not normally irritant to the average person. Common examples are metals (such as the nickel used in cheap jewellery), talcum powder and some foodstuffs.

Whichever form of eczema you suffer from, you will need to take special care with the type of products that you use on your scalp. Select a shampoo with as few colourings, perfumes and additives as possible, and take particular care to rinse the hair thoroughly.

If eczema is severe, special products can be used on the scalp, such as sulphur and salicylic acid in wax. You may also need to find out what foodstuffs provoke a reaction and eliminate these from your diet.

## SEBACEOUS CYSTS

The type known as trichilemmal cysts are the most common. These are round, smooth lumps, found either singly or in clusters on the scalp, and are formed in the outer root sheath of the hair follicle when keratin accumulates under the skin and forms a bump.

The cysts are completely harmless and only cause discomfort if they are accidentally damaged, perhaps by vigorous combing. If they become too big they can easily be removed under a local anaesthetic.

# Infections and infestations
# OF THE SCALP

**V**arious infections – boils, impetigo and ringworm – and infestations, most notably headlice, can affect the scalp.

## BOILS
This condition is caused by the common bacteria staphylococci invading a hair follicle or sebaceous gland and producing a severe inflammation, with swelling and pain.

## IMPETIGO
Impetigo is a streptococcal and/or staphylococcal infection and resembles tiny blisters filled with fluid, which form yellow crusts on the skin. It can occur as a result of scratching the scalp because of eczema or psoriasis, or because of a headlice infection.

## RINGWORM (TINEA)
This infection can occur anywhere on the skin or scalp and is caused by many different fungi. It results in bald (often circular) patches on the scalp, and the skin is usually inflamed. Ringworm is very itchy and highly infectious. It can be caught from cats, dogs and other domestic animals. The usual treatment is an anti-fungal agent, which is taken orally for a period of four to twelve weeks. Nizoral shampoo, which contains 2 per cent ketoconazole, may be used as well to help reduce the surface scaling.

## HEADLICE
Having headlice is nothing to be ashamed of, as an infestation affects most people at some point in their lives. At least 4 per cent of the population is infected by this tiny parasite at any one time, and it is extremely common in all young children who attend schools and

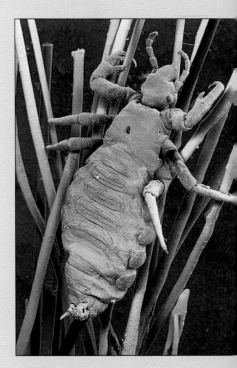

*Headlice are one of the most common parasites affecting both adults and children.*

nurseries. Cases have increased in recent years as the lice have developed immunity to the chemicals used to treat them. Headlice are tiny insects with flattened bodies, which live by sucking blood from the scalp. They lay their eggs (known as nits) on the base of the hairs, about 1cm/$\frac{1}{2}$in above the scalp, and are firmly glued into place. The larvae remain glued to the hair shaft and grow out with the hair. When a nit hatches out it must feed within 45 minutes if it is to survive. Headlice normally live for about 20–30 days and can lay 7–10 eggs per day during this time, so it does not take long for a couple of lice to become a major infection! They can survive for 24 hours away from the head, so may be transmitted via pillows, hats and towels, but are usually caught from direct head-to-head contact, as they cannot jump.

## TREATMENT

An infestation can easily be treated. Your pharmacist will provide a lotion containing a pesticide (usually malathion, carbaryl, permethrin or phenothrin). The current health-authority advice recommends personal rotation or the 'mosaic' method to reduce resistance. This means using the lotion once, then again in seven days' time. If a re-infestation occurs, repeat the procedure using a different chemical from last time, and so on until you return to the one you started with. The lotion should be applied to the hair and left for several hours (sometimes overnight). Lotions are more effective than the pesticide-containing shampoos, although the latter are more pleasant to use.

If you have young children who keep becoming infected with headlice, you can usually use the chemicals safely, if you do so as directed. Regular nit-combing is another safe and effective way of detecting and removing headlice, but it must be done thoroughly for several weeks to eliminate the lice completely.

## OTHER REMEDIES

A number of 'natural' remedies have been suggested, including lavender, tee-tree, geranium and olive oils. Most of these make the hair slippery, which aids in the removal of headlice. Other products contain alcohol, which may have some effect in stunning the lice and making them easier to comb out. None of these products, however, will kill the headlice or the eggs.

Electronic combs have now been developed to remove headlice, but their success has never been clinically proven.

# HOW TO USE A NIT-COMB

1 Select a very fine comb. Choose a plastic one, as metal damages the hair cuticle, but one that is very ridged, so that it will not give around the eggs.

2 Comb when the hair is wet, at three- to four-day intervals for 30 minutes, or every day if the infestation is severe.

3 If the hair is long or tends to tangle, use a conditioner to help the comb slide through it.

4 Carefully comb every area of the head, paying special attention to the nape of the neck and behind the ears.

5 Draw the comb firmly across the head close to the scalp, and then remove any lice from the comb.

# DANDRUFF

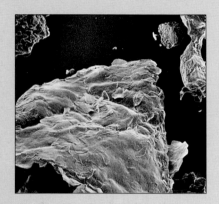

**O**ne hair problem that everyone worries about is dandruff – an umbrella term used for all forms of excessive scaling conditions, when pieces of skin appear on our hair and clothing. But it's important to realize that what we call dandruff is not always so! True dandruff is the condition also known as pityriasis capitis (see below).

Some loss of surface cells from the scalp is normal, as the uppermost skin cells die and are replaced by new ones from below. These scales are most conspicuous after hair has been brushed, since this can loosen the dead cells. Some people tend to have dry, flaky skin, and this may also cause a problem with scaling, especially if you wash your hair frequently. The washing removes the natural oils from the scalp, and the skin is shed in dry white flakes. When this is mistaken for dandruff, the hair is washed more often – sometimes with harsh shampoos – and the result is a vicious circle, with

the scalp becoming drier and drier. It may also become itchy, causing you to scratch and thus make the skin flake off more rapidly.

Eczema (see pp.68–9) can also affect the scalp, causing dry patches that may shed flakes of skin, which can be mistaken for dandruff. If you get eczema mainly on the scalp, you could be allergic to a particular ingredient in your shampoo, conditioner or colourant.

In seborrhoeic dermatitis, the layer of natural oil known as sebum, becomes crusty, dries out and is shed, causing unsightly sprinkling

## CURING DANDRUFF – 10 steps

Wash hair frequently using a mild shampoo.

**1**

If this doesn't work, try a specially formulated medicated shampoo.

**2**

Avoid scratching the scalp or combing it roughly.

**3**

Try anti-fungal agents on the scalp.

**4**

Try natural remedies, such as lemon juice or linseed oil rubbed into the scalp.

**5**

on the skin and clothes. Sometimes the scalp can become very irritated, with yellowish-red, greasy and scaly patches, especially along the hairline.

Pityriasis capitis is a condition in which a yeast known as Pityosporum ovale that lives on the skin and multiplies in the warm, moist, oily surface of the scalp, is sometimes (but not always) involved. It appears as white or grey scales (often 'dusty' in appearance), which may form small patches or cover the whole scalp. If the condition is as described, but oily, then the complaint may be pityriasis steatoides. If you have pityriasis, washing the hair every day with a mild, frequent-wash shampoo may solve the problem in a week or two. If this fails, try a proper anti-dandruff shampoo (not one that is simply adapted for frequent washing).

## MEDICATED SHAMPOOS

Some medicated shampoos act by stripping off the layer of dead skin and oil, which makes the hair look better at first, but does not attack the cause. Others that are not left on the scalp for long, will not attack the growth of the bacteria or yeast. Certain medicated shampoos contain the active ingredients zinc pyrithrone or selenium sulphide, which slow down cell growth on the scalp. Selenium also acts as an anti-fungal agent. It is important to follow the instructions carefully for these shampoos, as they can be toxic if overused. There are also anti-dandruff cleansing tonics or lotions that are left on the scalp long enough to kill off the offending bacteria.

## NATURAL REMEDIES

Some shampoos contain natural products, such as seaweed, sage and calendula, or citric acid. One natural remedy is simply to rub lemon juice into the scalp to create a very acid environment.

### HERBAL REMEDIES FOR DANDRUFF

100ml/3 1/2fl oz jojoba or apricot oil
20 drops orange oil
17 drops cedarwood oil
17 drops patchouli oil
10 drops tea-tree oil
Massage well into the scalp, cover hair with a towel and leave for a few hours, then shampoo out.

Or try sage or nettle oils massaged into the scalp each day and used warm as a final rinse when shampooing. Live natural yoghurt can also be placed on the scalp for 10 minutes, as an anti-fungal and anti-bacterial agent, before being rinsed off.

**6** Use clean towels to dry the hair and don't share or use damp towels.

**7** Try going on an 'anti-fungal diet' by cutting out refined sugars, carbohydrates, animal fats and hydrogenated margarines.

**8** Take supplements of zinc and vitamins B, C and E.

**9** Try supplements of oils that are high in polyunsaturates, such as cold-pressed sunflower and linseed oils.

**10** If dandruff is persistent, see a dermatologist.

# Unwanted hair

## AND DEPILATION

**W**hile women worry about their hair becoming thinner on their head, they frequently also worry about excess hair on the face, legs and body.

Some women have more body hair than others, and how visible it is will depend on its colour. Someone with plentiful blonde body hair may be far less troubled by it than someone with far less dark hair. While excessive facial hair is never acceptable in women, the extent to which women worry about hair under the arms or on their arms and legs varies in different cultures.

There are medical reasons why a woman may start to grow excessive facial or body hair. It can be a side-effect of oral contraceptives, danazol, cortisone and other steroids, and of the immuno-suppressant drug cyclosporin. In 5–10 per cent of patients, the anti-epilepsy drug phenytoin can also cause excessive hair growth; so can illnesses such as polycystic ovaries and disorders of the adrenal and pituitary glands. In these cases drugs may be used to alleviate the problem.

For most women, however, the problem is simply that they have more hair than they feel is compatible with the current ideal of beauty. They may deal with it by bleaching, depilation or epilation.

### BLEACHING
This is a very common method of making dark hairs less visible, and is often used on the face for a 'moustache' and on the arms and legs. The active ingredient is hydrogen peroxide (strengths above 6 per cent are not recommended), usually combined with ammonia to speed up its action and fragrances.

The bleach solution or powder is generally mixed with a paste to make it easier to apply, left on for a set amount of time, then rinsed off. Sometimes the skin is a little red afterwards but this should not last long. Bleaching also seems to act to soften the hairs, making them feel finer.

Some hair is more difficult to bleach and the product may need to be left on for longer than suggested, as long as this does not irritate the skin. However, if you leave it on for too long the hairs will be bleached too much, making them more obvious; there may also be a problem when the roots start to show colour.

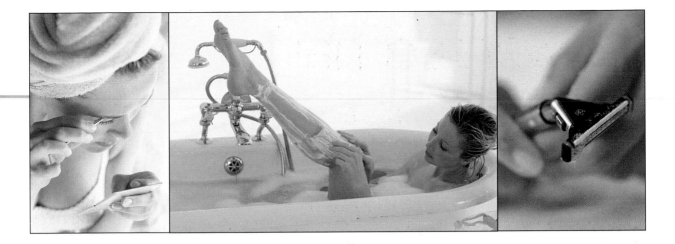

## METHODS OF HAIR REMOVAL:

■ **Depilation**

The hair is removed at the skinline; treatment is painless, but the hair soon grows back and may appear to be bristlier in texture. Depilation techniques include shaving and using depilatory creams that contain chemicals to dissolve the hair.

■ **Epilation**

The hair is removed from below the surface of the skin. The advantage is that the hair takes longer to grow back and the tip of the growing hair is finer than with depilation. Techniques include plucking with tweezers, waxing and electrolysis.

## SHAVING

Contrary to myth, shaving does not make your hair grow any faster, thicker or more dense. It simply removes the top portion of the hair where it emerges from the skin. After shaving, however, the hair growing back may look different because it has a thicker, blunter tip than ordinary hair.

Shaving is most commonly done on areas like the legs, and many women shave in the bath, because the hair is softened by soaking in the water. Use a lot of soap or foam to get a smoother shave. Standard safety razors give a closer shave than electric razors (which obviously must not be used in the bath). One disadvantage of shaving is that once you start you have to continue, sometimes as often as every day, to prevent stubble appearing. Apply plenty of moisturizer afterwards to avoid irritation to the skin.

## DEPILATORY CREAMS

The active ingredient in most depilatory creams is a salt of thioglycolic acid, usually calcium thioglycolate. These products do not smell pleasant, so a fragrance is usually added and sometimes a moisturizing cream. The thioglycolates break down the chemical bonds in the hair so that it becomes weak and finally disintegrates. These creams also penetrate a little below the surface of the hair follicle.

# EPILATION

Of the various epilatory techniques, plucking with tweezers is the simplest, but waxing and electrolysis are more effective.

## PLUCKING

This method is often used for removing small areas of hair, for instance around the eyebrows, on the upper lip and on the chin.

The problem with plucking is that when the hair is torn out from the follicle it can cause damage to the surrounding tissue, often resulting in sore red spots; on rare occasions, it can lead to long-term scarring, especially if the hair follicle becomes infected. To avoid this, careful cleaning of the skin before and after treatment is a good idea. Hairs that are constantly plucked may become coarser and darker than the original ones.

## WAXING

Waxing is probably the most effective method of removing unwanted hair in both small and large areas.

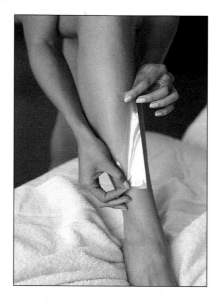

## COLD WAXING

This is the most common method used at home. Cold wax can be bought at most chemists and usually comes in tubes. The technique for using it is similar to that for warm waxing (see below), but the wax is usually applied to the skin with a tongue applicator and has a gauze or paper strip attached. Once the wax is cold, the strip is quickly ripped off against the direction of hair growth.

## WARM WAXING

This technique is more effective than cold waxing and is usually performed in a beauty salon. The wax is heated in a warmer until it has just melted and is then applied to the skin with a small wooden spatula. Next, a strip of cotton or muslin cloth is placed over the wax, which is allowed to cool. The strip is then quickly removed, being pulled in the opposite direction to the hair growth. Any discomfort is over within a few seconds. Hand pressure is then applied to the area in question to soothe it, although it may be red and sensitive for a few hours.

Sometimes alcohol is used to prevent any infection in the damaged hair follicles. The hair will not be visible for 10–14 days after waxing.

The follicles can become infected, and sometimes women experience problems with ingrowing hairs afterwards. These can be painful and liable to infection. Some women find the waxing procedure too painful to repeat, and a few feel really unwell afterwards, with sore, irritated skin.

## ELECTROLYSIS

Electrolysis is a permanent method of removing unwanted hairs by destroying the hair-growth tissue in the hair follicle.

A sterile needle or probe is inserted into the follicle and a small amount of electric current is then used to destroy the growing base of the hair. The hair is then removed with tweezers. Sometimes one treatment is enough to permanently stop the follicle producing hair. In other cases there is a regrowth, although often the new hair is finer than the original hair was.

All electrolysis equipment should be thoroughly sterilized to avoid the risk of infection. Many practitioners use pre-sterilized disposable needles, although others sterilize reusable needles. It's a good idea to discuss sterilization techniques with the beautician before you have any treatment. Make sure that the electrologist has a recognized diploma or certificate to show that they have been adequately trained.

The number of treatments depends on the individual. Deep, coarse hairs cannot usually be removed with one treatment. If you have been removing hair by plucking or with wax, then the hairs may be stronger and may require more treatments than hairs that have not previously been removed. The electrologist may take a few attempts to assess the right degree of current in order to remove hairs while causing the least pain and redness to the skin.

Electrolysis may be slightly – or uncomfortably – painful and feel like a mild burning or tingling sensation. Some parts of the body may be more sensitive than others. Depending on the amount of hair involved and its location, a session will usually last for a short enough time to keep discomfort down to an absolute minimum.

Immediately following treatment, there may be slight redness or swelling, which usually disappears in a few hours. Occasionally small whiteheads or tiny scabs may occur. These are part of the normal healing process and will not cause permanent damage or scarring, as long as they are not picked off. Electrolysis should not cause any lasting damage to the skin.

The downside of electrolysis is that it is time-consuming, because a limited number of hairs can be removed at each session. It is also expensive.

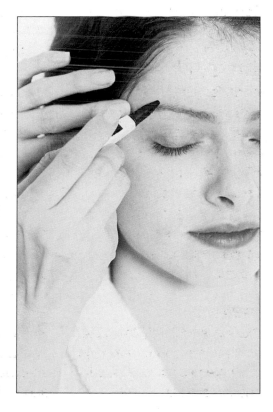

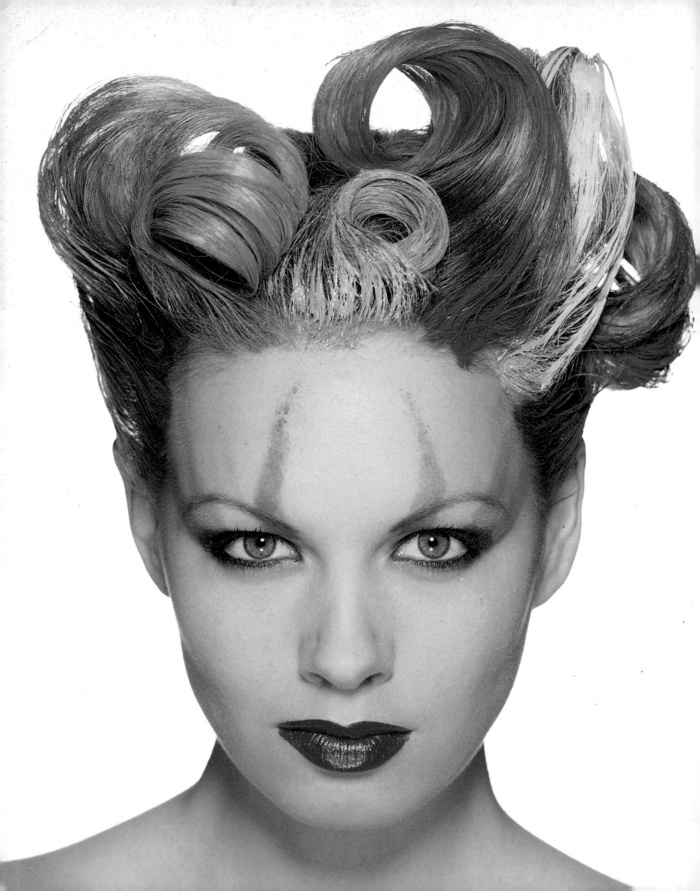

# HAIR
# Colour

# The range
# OF COLOURS

**H**air comes in a marvellous range of tones, from the palest blonde to jet-black or vibrant red, with every conceivable variation of shade in between.

## BLONDE
Blonde hair has always been prized, and it is often stated that 'gentlemen prefer blondes'. Many children are born with blonde hair, but this darkens as they age, so that blonde hair has always been linked with youth and innocence. Blonde has also been seen as the colour of sexual attractiveness, with generations of Hollywood stars bleaching their hair blonde to add glamour.

Blonde can vary in colour from almost white through to a rich, golden honey colour. Strawberry-blonde has a high proportion of red hairs mixed in. The sun has a natural bleaching effect on the hair, so blonde hair also acts in the same way as a suntan to enhance attractiveness. Women with light brown or mousy hair often develop natural blonde highlights in the summer and it is easy to tint the hair to enhance and re-create this effect.

## BRUNETTE
Brown hair can come in any shade from mousy through to a rich, deep chestnut brown – or even verging on pure black. Often brown hair has different layers of tone in it, which lends it depth and movement. Brown hair may accompany many different tones of skin, from pale to deep olive, which gives it different effects. This is the most versatile of all hair

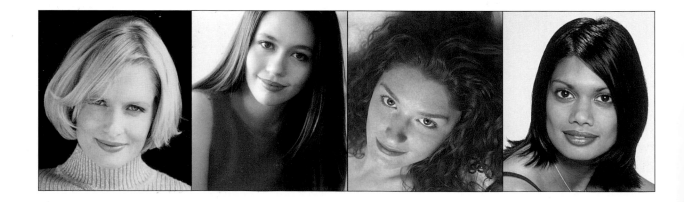

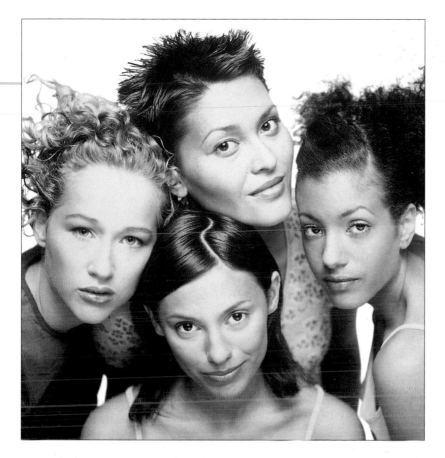

portraits of women with long Titian tresses. Today red hair has become fashionable again and many women want to tint or dye their hair one of the glorious shades of red.

## BLACK

Black hair can glow and shine like no other – 'like a raven's wing', as it is described in many fairy stories. Snow White, with her white skin, red lips and jet-black hair, was an ideal of beauty. Oriental women have straight black hair, which is thick and strong and can be grown longer than any other kind of hair without splitting or becoming damaged at the ends.

colours and the easiest to tint, highlight or colour Because it comes in the middle of the colour chart, it is easy to go either way – to lighten hair to blonde, to darken it or to add rich red tones.

## REDHEAD

Historically, red hair was regarded as dangerous and, perhaps because red hair was so rare, redheads were often stigmatized and believed to be witches or in league with the Devil. They were viewed as wicked and ill-tempered, and the Romans found the red-headed warriors of ancient Britain fierce enemies. This reputation continued, and in works of art from AD1300 onwards Judas was often portrayed with red hair.

In the 1500s Elizabeth I made red hair fashionable in England, and in the late nineteenth century Pre-Raphaelite painters gloried in

Afro hair has its own beauty, with its thick, magnificent curliness. It is extremely versatile and permits a variety of styles. In mixed-race people, the tight curliness of African Caribbean hair may be combined with other hair types and colours, and it can be tinted and lightened just like any other hair. Mixed-race hair may grow longer than pure-Afro hair, giving long curly locks that can look wonderful.

# What causes
# HAIR COLOUR?

Natural hair colour is determined by the presence of pigments in the hair shaft. The most common pigment is the black or brown melanin, while red and yellow hair is produced by a pigment called pheomelanin. In colours in between there is a mixture of both pigments in the hair. The amount of pigment determines the darkness and depth of the colour. The pigment is found mainly in the cortex, with a small amount in the cuticle. Melanin molecules are granular in appearance, while pheomelanin molecules are small and scattered, and there are more of them. Pigments work by absorbing certain wavelengths or colours in the light and reflecting others. White hair has no pigment and reflects all light, whereas black hair absorbs light of every wavelength.

## THE GENETIC LINK

Your hair colour is pre-determined at birth and is inherited from your parents, although you won't always have the same colour hair as they do. This is because of the way inherited characteristics are passed on in the genes.

If you inherit a gene for black hair from your mother and blonde hair from your father, then since you can't have both colours of hair, one gene is dominant over the other. Black hair is dominant over blonde, which is dominant over red.

When an inherited characteristic is 'dominant', this means that it always shows and that any other inherited gene is masked. However, the masked gene is still present and may combine with other genes in your children to express itself later. For example, you and your partner might both have black or brown hair, but be carrying a masked gene for red hair. If your child inherits both genes for red hair, you will have an unexpected redhead in the family.

## LINKS TO SKIN TYPE

Your hair colour is also closely related to your skin colour. On the whole, the darker the hair colour, the darker the skin. Thus black-skinned women almost always have black hair, while pale blondes have fair skin, and redheads have the palest skin of all, because their skin contains so little melanin. An exception to this is the striking Celtic combination of pale (sometimes freckled) skin and deep brown or black hair. Very rarely, dark-skinned people of mixed race can have blonde or red hair.

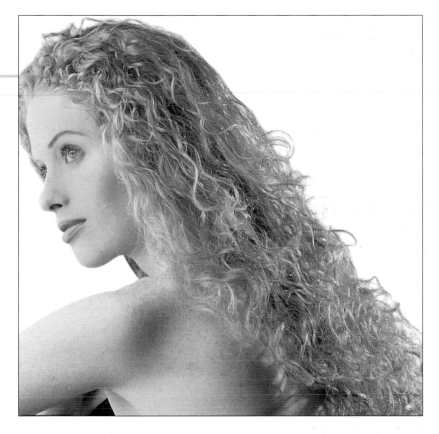

Albinos are people whose bodies lack the normal pigments, melanin and pheomelanin. Their skins are extremely pale, their eyes are pink and their hair is completely white. Albino people can be of any race, and the gene for this is recessive, so that the parents of albino children may have normal colouring. If an albino person marries someone with normal colouring, their children will not be albinos (although they will carry the recessive gene).

## HAIR COLOURING THROUGH THE AGES

Since the dawn of civilization women have used natural herbs and chemicals to change the colour of their hair. Roman women used concoctions of wood ash, sodium bicarbonate and unslaked lime to lighten their hair, and copper filings mixed with oak-apples to darken it. The Teutons in Germany used lead oxide, ochre and vermilion with soap to form 'Sapo', which cleansed the hair and coloured it red.

In Turkey, during the Constantine Empire, women used gall-oak, mixed with oil and white lead, to form a blackening paste, while during the Renaissance women bleached their hair with a blend of borax and saltpetre. Saffron, mullein and exotic myrrh were also used to tint the hair. To obtain the Titian colour so admired at that time, they applied a paste of ashes and herbs. Sulphur, alum and honey were also used.

Hydrogen peroxide, the base of most modern bleaches and permanent hair colourants, was discovered in 1818 and first used in 1860 by Napoleon II's mistress, Cora Pearl. At about the same time coal-tar dyes were discovered by the German chemist Wilhelm von Hofman and his student, William Henry Peck, at London's Royal College of Chemistry. Von Hofman was trying to synthesize quinine, but ended up with a dark sludge, which, when diluted with alcohol, turned purple. These coal-tar dyes form the base of the chemical colourants used today.

# Choosing a
# HAIR COLOUR

Changing the colour of your hair can transform your appearance, making you look younger and more attractive. There are three main ways you can change your hair: by choosing a striking new colour – going blonde from brunette, or going red; by subtly lightening or darkening your natural colour; and by covering up grey. Sometimes a dramatic change in cut – from long hair to short, or a complete change of style – will look better with a change in hair colour, too.

Today it is much easier to change the colour of your hair, with new products that can help you tint your hair at home or in the salon. Colours have become more subtle, often mixed with natural ingredients, and a far wider variety of products can help you find the right type and colour for your hair.

It helps to start with the advice of a hairdresser and to try out new colours in the salon. Once you have found a product that works for you, you may then feel confident about using it at home. Some colour treatments, such as highlights, are always best done by a skilled hairdresser, as the effect can be hard to achieve yourself.

Certain treatments, especially those that lighten the hair, may cause some damage to it, which may be cumulative. So if your hair is very dark there will be a limit to the amount of time you can stay ash-blonde (and, of course, ash-blonde colouring will be more difficult to achieve in the first place if your hair is very dark). In between, you may need to try other styles and colours; having your hair cut short can get around the problem when you are growing it out after a

dramatic colour change, and you can use a temporary colour to cover the hair while a permanent tint grows out.

**MATCHING HAIR TO SKIN TONE**

Choosing the right colour for your hair can be difficult, especially the first time you try something new. The most important thing is to take account of your skin tone, to make sure that the colour will look natural on you. This is especially important as you age, as the skin tends to get paler as you grow older, and dark hair that looked stunning in your 20s can look too harsh when you reach your 50s.

Holding a card with the potential hair colour on up to the face – rather as you might hold up material for a dress – so that the colour reflects on your skin, can help. It is important to do this in daylight rather than the artificial light of a salon. Often a contrast looks good; skin that is red in tone will look redder with red or auburn hair and may look better with dark, more blueish-tinted hair. When a woman starts to go grey, her skin colour often lightens, so colours that looked good when she was younger may now be too hard. Highlighting, or colouring only some of the hair, may produce a more subtle effect.

### USING SUBTLE COLOUR CHANGES

Colouring your hair close to your natural shade is much easier and helps prevent problems as hair grows out. Hair grows at an average of 1.25cm ($1/2$in) a month, so women who go dramatically blonde may have to have their roots retinted as often as every four to six weeks. With highlights (see pp.98–99), it may be eight weeks or more before the difference shows.

As hair turns grey, it is easy to cover up the first few white hairs with a colour close to your natural colour. Often a semi-permanent colour will be satisfactory. However, as hair becomes greyer, disguising the root regrowth will become more and more of a problem. Again, using highlights can help make the change more gradual and create a more subtle and natural effect.

Remember that when you change your hair colour, you may have to change your wardrobe and make-up, too. Lipsticks that looked great with your old brunette hair may clash dreadfully with your new strawberry-blonde, and the same may apply to your favourite scarlet dress.

## BEST COLOUR COMBINATIONS

| | SKIN TONE | COLOUR CHOICE |
|---|---|---|
| 1 | Pale or ivory | Any hair colour will look good when young; when older, avoid too dark or intense colours. |
| 2 | Rosy | Avoid red or golden-blonde; choose ash tones to neutralize your skin tone. |
| 3 | Yellow | Avoid yellow, gold or orange; go for deep reds and rich burgundies. |
| 4 | Olive | Stay dark, adding richness; warm chestnut or burgundy will look good. |

# TYPES OF hair colouring

Hair colourants come in three main types: temporary, semi-permanent and permanent. In fact the division between the three is not quite so clear-cut, with different products filling in the gaps.

## TEMPORARY COLOURS

Temporary hair colours are water-based and simply sit on the outside of the hair, rinsing out with each wash (or lasting at most for a couple of washes).

## SEMI-PERMANENT COLOURS

Semi-permanent colours sit both on the outside of the cuticle (the outer layer of the hair) and also penetrate slightly under the cuticle to colour the hair more permanently. These colours will usually stay on the hair for between four and six washes, as long as the hair is not bleached by the sun or chlorine, which will cause it to fade faster.

These colours last longer than temporary colours but not as long as permanent dyes,

lasting for six to eight washes. They are unlikely to cause damage to the hair, or affect perming or the use of more permanent colours later. They are resistant to brushing and shampooing.

## PERMANENT COLOURS

A full tint or permanent hair colour contains an activator that opens the hair and allows the colour in under the cuticle, penetrating the cortex and then enabling the cuticle to close again, trapping the colour inside. The tint stays there until it grows out, although it may fade a little in the sun or after swimming in a chlorinated pool.

## NATURAL COLOURANTS

Concern about using chemicals on the hair, and the effects this may have on the hair itself (and on the skin, if absorbed through the scalp into the body) have led to new, organic or natural hair colourants being developed. These use natural herb extracts to colour the hair, either in shampoos or in colourings. Herbal extracts

include walnut (which contains the natural colourant juglone) for dark brown or black hair, and chamomile (which contains apigenine) to lighten blonde or light brown hair. Cornflower can be used for its blue pigment (cyanocentaurine), which can give an attractive silver colour to white or grey hair.

## HENNA

The henna plant contains a natural pigment called lawsone and henna has long been used as a natural hair colourant. While it gives a rich colour to brown or chestnut hair, the effect on blonde or grey hair can be startlingly bright. Henna also coats the hair, sticking strongly to the outside of the cuticle, strengthening it and giving it body, but also tending to prevent moisture and conditioning products getting into the hair, which may make it dry. Because henna coats the surface of the hair so thickly, hair that has been hennaed will not take another pigment until the henna has been allowed to grow out.

# THE INTERNATIONAL COLOURING SYSTEM

To help the consumer or hairdresser, hair colours are described in terms of depth and tone. Depth describes how dark or light the colour is, and tone is the colour you see (i.e. the combination of pigments). Warm shades, such as gold or red, have more red and yellow pigments, while cool shades such as ash have fewer. The International Colouring System defines hair colour and should be displayed on most hair colourants. Shades are divided and numbered as below:

| DEPTH | TONE |
| --- | --- |
| 1/0 blue-black | 0 natural |
| 2/0 black | 1 ash |
| 3/0 dark brown | 2 cool ash |
| 4/0 medium brown | 3 honey-gold |
| 5/0 light brown | 4 red |
| 6/0 dark blonde | 5 purple |
| 7/0 medium blonde | 6 violet |
| 8/0 light blonde | 7 brunette |
| 9/0 very light blonde | 8 pearl ash |
| 10/0 extra light blonde | 9 soft ash |

This means that a colour with, say, 6/1 will be dark blonde (depth) with ash (tone).

# THE PRINCIPLES of colour

If you are thinking about colouring your hair, it helps to understand how colours work and mix together.

The three primary colours – colours that cannot be made by mixing other colours – are red, blue and yellow. All other colours are created by mixing these colours together: red and blue to make purple; blue and yellow to make green; and red and yellow to make orange. Mixing all three primary colours together evenly makes black, while mixing them in different proportions can make brown. Some colours are complementary to one another; in other words, these colours tend to 'neutralize' each other. For instance, orange is neutralized by blue; yellow by purple or mauve.

Understanding these principles is important when choosing a colourant for your hair. If your hair is yellowish, for example, and you use a blue rinse, then your hair will tend towards green. This can be avoided by adding a red toner. If your hair has a lot of red in it, adding a yellowish colour will make it tend towards orange. Adding a blue toner can eliminate this problem.

**TEMPORARY COLOURS**

These are useful for people who may want to try out new hair colours on a temporary basis before committing themselves, or who may want to change their hair colour for some special occasion. They are also used by fashion models to create stunning effects for a photo session. They usually wash out completely the next time you shampoo your hair, so if you make a terrible mistake it is quickly and easily put right. If,

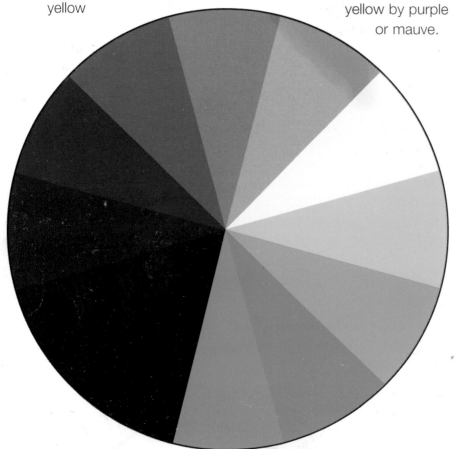

*The colour wheel shows the complete range of colours.*

however, your hair is very porous, then the colour may get inside the cuticle of the hair and last for one or two more washes. This can be useful when older women use a tint to cover up grey hairs or to take the yellow shades out of white hair.

Temporary colourants are also used in some mousses, gels, hair sprays and shampoos. You can also buy coloured sprays and 'hair mascaras' to tint the hair when it is dry and to create effects for a party or special occasion.

Overuse of temporary colours can produce a build-up of colour, which may dull the hair. It may also have a more permanent effect on porous hair (such as previously bleached, permed or long hair), as the pigment can enter the hair shaft.

## SEMI-PERMANENT COLOURS

These colours are bought ready to use, require no mixing and are easy to apply. They are usually put on to freshly shampooed hair that has been dabbed dry with a towel. They are normally left on the hair for about 10–30 minutes and then rinsed off. They can be applied with a tint brush or sponge, or simply massaged directly into the hair. They work through some of the colour molecules penetrating under the cuticle of the hair and remaining in the cortex. The molecules of pigment have to be fairly small to allow this to happen, and the product has to have a pH of between 8 and 9 (that is, quite alkaline) to help open the cuticle and enable this to happen. Semi-permanent colours are used to add tones to hair colour, such as gold, ash, copper or burgundy; to darken the hair and effectively cover up to 30 per cent of white hair; to disguise unwanted colours, such as a yellowish tinge to white hair; and to brighten and enhance hair colour generally. They cannot lighten hair colour.

Semi-permanents generally come as liquids and creams, non-drip foams and mousses; they can also be used in shampoos. They are easy to apply at home and do not normally cause allergies.

# The most commonly used ingredients:

| 1 | 2 | 3 | 4 | |
|---|---|---|---|---|
| **SODIUM BISULPHIDE** | **HYDROGEN PEROXIDE** | **NITRO-PHENYLENEDIAMINES** | **ANTHRAQUINONES** | Permanent oxidation tints include combinations of different chemicals, including para-phenylenediamines (black), para-toluenediamines (brown), meta-hydroxybenzine (grey), para-aminiophenol (reddish-brown) and meta-phenylenediamines (brown). |
| A reducing agent used to strip colour, especially old colourants, from the hair. Bleach is also used in a weak form for this purpose. | An oxidizing agent used to bleach hair. It is used with all semi-permanent colourants to open up the cuticle and allow the colourant in. | The most predominant semi-permanent colourings that give red and yellow colours. | The main semi-permanent colourings that give blue colours. | |

# PERMANENT COLOURS and bleaches

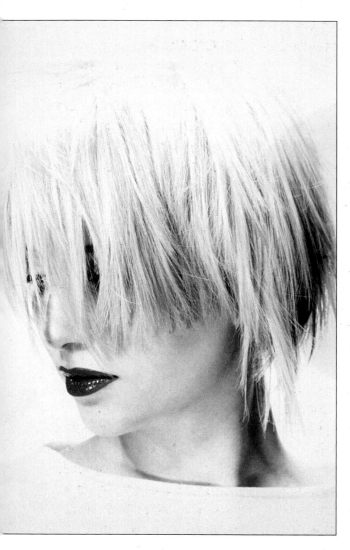

Colourants that give a more permanent effect fall into two categories: quasi-permanent and permanent.

## QUASI-PERMANENT COLOURS

These are non-lightening colours that are mixtures of the dyes used in semi-permanents and permanents, and require mixing with an oxidation agent such as hydrogen peroxide, though in lower concentration than is needed for permanent hair colours.

In these colours, the hydrogen peroxide content is only about 1–3 per cent and is often called a 'colour activator', 'colour releaser' or 'colour developer'. The oxidant acts to lock the colours inside the cuticle, but, because the hydrogen peroxide is of such a low strength, it does not affect the natural colour of your hair. The colour will fade a little each time you wash it, but a permanent change of colour will also become visible at the roots. Because quasi-permanents contain some of the permanent dyes, a skin test (see p.93) is always necessary before using one.

This kind of colour can be used to add shine and to enhance natural hair colour, to cover up to 50 per cent of white hairs and to refresh old highlights. Quasi-permanent usually come as creams or liquids that become gel-like when mixed with the oxidant.

## PERMANENT COLOURS

These are the only colourants that will completely cover hair, including 100 per cent of white hair, in any colour shade. They must all be used with hydrogen peroxide, which enables the colour to penetrate inside the cuticle of the hair.

Permanent tints are applied to dry, unwashed hair after a skin test has been carried out. Oxidation tints must be applied carefully to the hair with a brush to ensure that the tint is applied only to the right parts of the hair. This is particularly important if the tint is for a regrowth. Since a noticeable regrowth is apparent after four to six weeks, frequent retouching is needed.

The pH of oxidation tints is 8.5–9.5, and this opens the cuticle and allows penetration of the colourant. The tint usually takes 30–45 minutes to develop, during which time the molecules of dye come together to form larger molecules that cannot then escape from the cortex.

Permanent hair colours enable you to choose whatever shade of hair you want, no matter what your age or the natural colour of hair. They are also used to disguise white hair completely and to lighten or darken hair. They can simultaneously bleach and colour. However, the use of hydrogen peroxide can damage your hair if used too often.

Most of these colourants come as liquids, creams and oils, which gel when added to the oxidant. The strength of the hydrogen peroxide ranges from 3 to 12 per cent. Higher-strength peroxide is sometimes needed to lighten colour.

## BLEACHING

Bleaching is the removal of natural hair colour. The bleaching agent oxidizes the molecules of the natural pigments, melanin and pheomelanin, to produce the colourless oxymelanin.

Pheomelanins will only react to the bleach after all the melanin that is present has been removed. If the melanin is not entirely removed, then the phcomelanin will remain intact. This reaction enables the hairdresser to control the colour of the hair as it bleaches, stopping the process at the appropriate point to obtain the desired effect. Bleaching can also be done to lighten the hair before adding another colour to it.

Bleaching is normally done using hydrogen peroxide with another oxidant and a catalyst to speed up the reaction. Bleaches may come as a powder or paste, an oil or an emulsion, and can also be found in lightening shampoos and setting lotions.

## POWDER BLEACH

This can lift hair colour by four to six shades. It consists of ammonium carbonate and magnesium carbonate. This is mixed with hydrogen peroxide to make a smooth paste that is thin enough to be applied to the hair but thick enough not to run. Some people may experience a tightening or burning sensation on their scalp when using a powder bleach, in which case another type of bleach may be preferable.

## EMULSION BLEACH

This contains potassium persulphate or ammonium persulphate and can lighten hair by six shades. Antiseptic conditioning agents, such as cetrimide, are sometimes added to help reduce damage to the hair.

## OIL BLEACH

This is a soluble oil mixed with hydrogen peroxide to form a transparent gel that is easy to apply. Oil bleaches can only lift hair colour by two or three shades.

# Steps to a
# NEW COLOUR

If you are thinking of changing your hair colour, it can help to try a temporary colour first (see pp.88–89), to see what the effect is. You can easily use these colourants at home and there is no danger of doing any damage to your hair.

## TIPS IF YOU ARE TINTING YOUR HAIR AT HOME

- Protect your skin: rub Vaseline on to your hairline to prevent staining and always wear rubber gloves.

- Always follow the instructions on the packet to the letter.

- If the packet gives timing guidelines, have a reliable clock to hand and stick to that timing exactly. Not doing so can cause damage to your hair or skin.

If you decide you want a more permanent colour, it is advisable to go to a good hair salon. The hairdresser will discuss the different options available, will examine your hair to see what kind of treatment is best suited to you, and will do tests to make sure that you do not develop an allergic reaction to any of the hair products.

## STRAND TEST

Before colouring your hair, you or the hairdresser should always test the colour on an individual strand of hair. This is especially important if your hair has been coloured or bleached before. A strand test will help monitor colour development and will show you what the final colour of your hair will be.

A strand of hair is taken and the product applied, then the hair is wrapped in foil until the colour has developed. The product is removed with damp cotton wool and the hair examined to check whether the colour has developed evenly.

A hairdresser will also test the porosity of the hair, to see how quickly and easily it will take the dye. If the hair is damaged, the cuticle will be rough and more porous, letting large quantities of dye into the hair quickly. The colour may also fade faster afterwards. The porosity is indicated by the roughness of the individual hairs, so a hairdresser will take strands of your hair at different points on the scalp and run her fingers over them to see how rough they feel. The resulting porosity will affect how long the colourant is left to work.

The elasticity of the hair can also be tested to see if hair is damaged. The hairdresser takes an individual hair and pulls it to see how far it stretches and springs back. The less elastic the hair, the more damaged – and therefore the more porous – it will be.

## SKIN TEST

A skin test should always be done before quasi-permanent or permanent colours are applied, to check that they will not irritate the scalp. First, you are protected by a gown and towel, then a small area of skin behind the ear, or on the inside of the elbow, is wiped with surgical spirit and the tint and hydrogen peroxide are applied to it. The area is allowed to dry and then covered with a colourless liquid called collodion, which will produce a clear layer over it. If a reaction develops there over the next 24 hours, then the product should not be used.

It is possible to become allergic to an unaltered product after years of use, and for a reaction suddenly to take place, so it may be worth doing a skin test before colouring, even if you have used the same product without problems many times before.

The most common allergies are to the para-dyes contained in oxidation tints. Para-phenylenediamine causes the largest number of reactions, in about one in 25 people. Such products are banned in Germany, Austria and France, although these countries still manufacture the dyes for use elsewhere. Research has shown that in large quantities they cause cancer in laboratory animals, but this has not been demonstrated in humans. However, they are unlikely to cause harm in the quantities used by most people, or even by the hairdresser.

Very rarely these products can cause severe allergic reactions, resulting in breathing difficulties and admission to hospital. If you have never used one of these products before, it is essential to have a skin test done.

## INCOMPATIBILITY TEST

Hairdressers will also carry out an incompatibility test to check whether any products that you have previously used on your hair will react badly with the planned tint or colourant. This specifically tests for the metallic salts contained in some henna products and colour restorers. Hydrogen peroxide reacts violently with these metallic salts and can damage both hair and scalp.

# AFTER COLOUR CARE and using henna

The process of colouring hair often irritates the scalp and disturbs its pH (acidity or alkalinity, see p.32); causes the cuticle layer to open, resulting in a loss of moisture from the hair; and disturbs the inner parts of the hair. And when the tint is rinsed out, stray oxidants are often left behind, which will cause the colour to fade if they are not neutralized.

Shampoos with a low pH (4.5–5.5) are most suitable for bleached or tinted hair because they help reduce the oxidation damage and close the cuticle, so that fewer colour molecules can escape and there is less fading.

## SHAMPOOS FOR USE ON TINTED HAIR

These often contain:

- Antioxidants

- UV filters to protect the hair from the bleaching effect of the sun

- Moisturizing agents to conserve moisture, smooth the cuticles and combat static

- Proteins or silicones to make hair easier to comb, and to add strength, texture and body

- A milder cleansing base than ordinary shampoos.

## USING HENNA

Henna has been used to add natural organic colour and shine to hair since antiquity. It comes from the dried leaves of the privet *Lawsonia alba* which grows in northern Africa and Asia. The active ingredient is lawsone, which was isolated in 1709 by the famous botanist Dr Israel Lawson. The leaves are harvested, dried in the sun and then crushed to a green powder. If the leaves are collected before they are fully mature, the product is green henna, which produces a more delicate shade of red with a slight yellow tone. Fully mature henna produces a rich red. Indigo is sometimes

## How to apply henna:

| 1 | 2 | 3 | 4 | 5 | 6 |
|---|---|---|---|---|---|
| First, wash and shampoo the hair, then towel it dry. | Smear a barrier cream round the ears and hairline, as henna stains the skin. Wear thin gloves if your hands will be in contact with the henna for long. | Apply the paste with a brush from the roots of the hair to the ends. | Leave the hair for the length of time required – just 10 minutes will give a red tint to pale hair, but several hours may be required to colour dark hair. | Keep the hair wrapped up in a towel or cap while the colour is developing to conserve moisture. | Rinse the henna off and shampoo several times to remove all traces of it from the hair and scalp. |

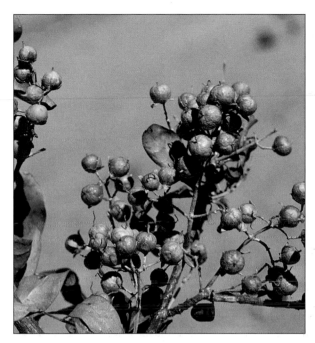

*The leaves of* Lawsonia alba *are dried and crushed to produce a form of henna that can be used as a dye.*

mixed with henna to produce Persian henna, which dyes the hair blue-black. Neutral henna is obtained from the root of the plant and is used for conditioning purposes rather than colouring.

Henna actually coats the cuticle of the hair, rather than getting inside. The colour fades gradually over six to eight weeks, so that you do not get a harsh line as it grows out. When henna is applied to brown or black hair you get a warm, reddish glow, while lighter hair goes a reddish-gold. It is definitely not suitable for white hair as it can go an intense orange. Henna is sometimes mixed with metallic salts to produce a full range of colours. This type of henna cannot be mixed with, or used after, any product that contains hydrogen peroxide, or a chemical reaction will take place that can severely damage the hair. If you are in any doubt about what kind of henna you have used, it is essential to have a strand test to check for metal deposits before having any perming, tinting or colouring done.

Natural henna is normally mixed to a smooth paste with hot water. Using milk can give it a creamier consistency, which is easy to use. Red wine can give a deeper tone, while adding coffee gives a beautiful chestnut brown, which can be especially useful on greying hair.

Henna is non-toxic, non-irritating to the skin and adds shine and body to the hair; it can also sometimes help to clear up dandruff. However, it can gradually dry the hair if used too often. Washing and general weathering will cause henna to fade, but it can only be removed entirely by allowing it to grow out. While this is happening it may be difficult, or impossible, to use other tints or colours on the hair.

### REMOVING HENNA BUILD-UP

If you have a build-up of henna on the hair after several applications, you can try removing it with a mixture of alcohol and mineral oil:

- Use 70 per cent alcohol to 30 per cent mineral oil and mix together well.

- Apply from the roots to the ends and leave on hair for 30 minutes.

- Rinse away the residue.

- You may need to do this two or three times.

# OTHER vegetable dyes

The following natural dyes coat the hair rather than entering the hair shaft. You can use them at home and you don't need to do a skin test first. However, you do have to use them regularly in order to keep up the effect.

### CHAMOMILE

This contains a yellow colourant, which, when infused and used on mousy or lighter-coloured hair, gives a lightening effect, by coating the hair with a yellow pigment, although it cannot actually lighten the hair. To make an infusion, use two tablespoons of fresh herbs and 600ml (1 pint) of boiling water, or make a paste with two tablespoons of dried flower heads and two tablespoons of kaolin, mixed with water to form a smooth consistency. Apply chamomile as you would henna (see page 94).

### SAGE

This herb darkens the hair, and an infusion is generally used on grey hair in order to tone the colour to a more silvery hue.

### RHUBARB ROOT

This will lighten brown bases and give golden highlights, if the application is followed by a spell in the sun. Boil a handful of rhubarb roots in water for one hour, then cool and strain the liquid. Use it as

*Marigolds give a yellow tinge to the hair, while sage will darken the hair.*

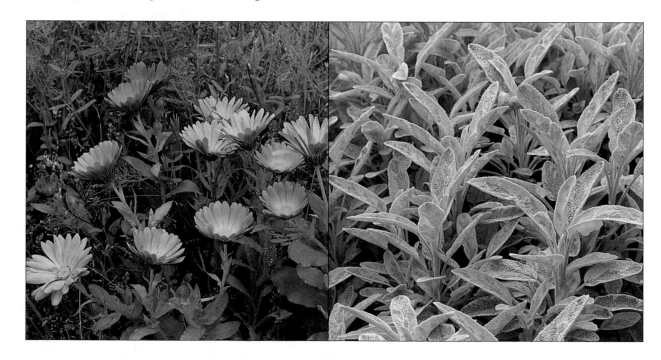

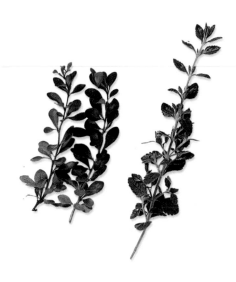

## QUASSIA

This is a tree bark that is often used in conjunction with chamomile to brighten the hair.

## CASCARILLA

Cascarilla is a tree bark that produces a strong black dye, which can be used to give brown tones to grey hair. The bark should be infused, cooled and then used as a final rinse.

## WALNUTS

Walnuts can be used to darken hair. To make the dye, boil the unripened green shells in water for two hours, then strain and cool the liquid. Use it as a final rinse.

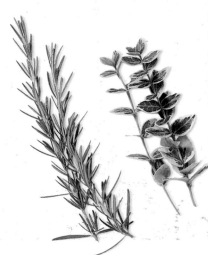

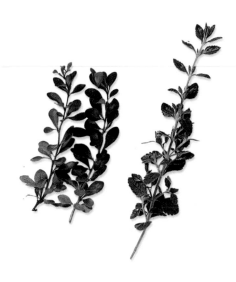

a final rinse after shampooing your hair. Rhubarb root can, however, leave a yellowish tinge on blonde or white hair.

## MARIGOLD

This gives a weaker yellow tinge to hair. Again, an infusion can be used as a final rinse.

## SAFFRON

Saffron is made from the dried stigmas of *Crocus sativus*. It gives bright yellow hues to natural blonde, tinted or bleached hair. Boil a few strands of saffron in 600ml (1 pint) of water, then dilute and use as a final rinse.

## 'NATURAL' HAIR COLOURANTS

Recently, permanent hair colours have been developed that claim to use natural dyes, but are also mixed with hydrogen peroxide to enable them to penetrate the hair cuticle. However, many of these products contain natural ingredients simply in addition to the usual chemicals in hair dyes, so skin tests should always be carried out before using them. It is important to read the list of ingredients and instructions before using this kind of product, or check with your hairdresser to see how they should be used. Frequent use can result in the hair becoming extremely dry and porous.

# Highlights
# AND LOWLIGHTS

**H**ighlighting and lowlighting are techniques for lightening and darkening selected strands of hair by using a cap or plastic bag, foil or clingfilm to cover most hair while the remaining hairs are being treated. During highlighting, the selected hair is bleached or coloured a lighter colour; while during lowlighting it is darkened, creating the opposite effect. Highlighting is best carried out by a skilled hairdresser as it is difficult to do yourself.

## HIGHLIGHTING

Highlights can make either a subtle or a dramatic difference to the colour of your hair, depending on how much hair is coloured and how different that colour is. It often looks more natural than tinting the whole head and it takes longer for the different colour at the roots to become noticeable, so they do not have to be retouched every six weeks or so – in fact, three months may go by before the hair needs treatment again. Highlighting often imitates the natural bleaching effect of the sun in summer or the mixture of different colours in a head of hair, so it has a less artificial look. The tint used should be at least two shades lighter than the natural colour to produce an overall lightening effect. One to three colours can be used to create the effect of different shades in natural hair.

## LOWLIGHTING

Lowlights are used on fine streaks of hair to produce a natural effect. This technique is particularly useful on grey hair, as lowlights blend the white hairs with the natural-coloured hair. Lowlighting can also produce good results on bleached or very light hair, putting darker toning lights into it. Again, more than one colour can be blended in the hair to produce a subtle result.

## Tips for highlighting and lowlighting:

| 1 | 2 | 3 | 4 |
|---|---|---|---|
| It is often best to start with subtle coloration and become more adventurous when you have got used to the effect. | When a subtle effect is required, look at the natural colours in your hair and emphasize these, rather than introducing foreign colours. | Do not use too bright or too dark colours if you are older, as these can look harsh. | It is better to have too few highlights than too many. If you don't have enough, you can always add more, but it is harder to remove highlights. |

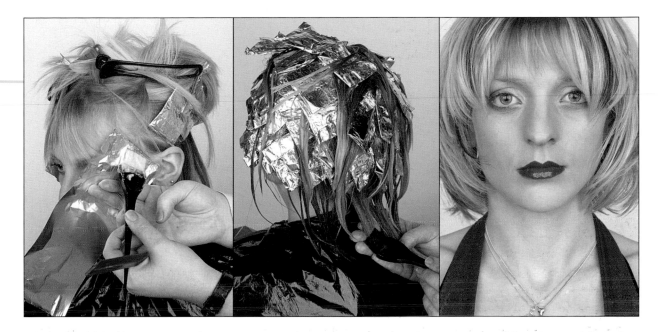

*The hair to be highlighted is separated out, wrapped in foil and the colourant applied with a brush.*

*The tint is left on the hair long enough for the colour to develop.*

*The final result is often a more natural look than an all-over bleach.*

### THE CAP METHOD

In this method the head is covered with a rubber or plastic cap and fine strands of hair are pulled through tiny holes with a crochet hook. It is not suitable for long hair. It is vital that the holes do not become too big and that the bleach or colourant forms a stiff enough paste not to run down through the holes and under the cap.

Nowadays the cap method is not used so often as most hairdressers prefer to use the foil method.

### THE FOIL METHOD

This method takes more time and effort, but it produces a more subtle effect. The hair is sectioned first to make it easier to work quickly, with the hairdresser usually dividing the head into six sections or more.

The bleach or colourant is woven in and out of the hair, and each tinted section is then wrapped in foil to form a parcel, so that the tint does not come into contact with the rest of the hair. Speed is essential so that some parts of the hair are not treated for longer than others, creating an uneven effect. The foil parcels are then removed in the same order as they were put in so that the dyes or bleaches are left on the hair for the same length of time.

When the effect starts to grow out, more highlights and lowlights can be added at the root ends of the hair. Because fewer hairs are treated, highlighting and lowlighting should cause little damage to the hair.

# Colouring African Caribbean
## AND GREY HAIR

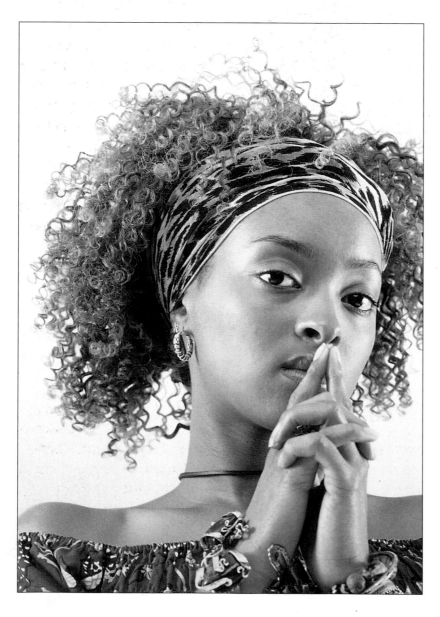

**A**frican Caribbean hair can be successfully coloured and tinted, although the hair almost invariably has to be lightened since it is dark to begin with. Too much bleaching will obviously cause damage to the hair, and temporary colours are not usually effective, because the hair underneath is too dark for them to show, although they can be used successfully to mask grey hairs.

When white women dye their hair black to cover grey hairs, this often looks harsh, because the skin becomes paler as they age. Black and Asian women, though, can get away with dyeing their hair black for longer as they grow older, because the black hair goes more successfully with their darker skin tone. However, silvery highlights can also look good on black hair.

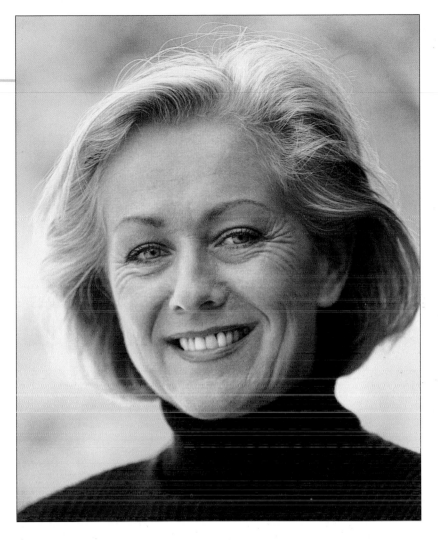

women develop a white streak in their hair in one location before the rest of the head develops any white hairs at all.

Grey hair is an obvious – and highly visible – sign of age, and today most women choose to disguise this. Colouring the hair is easy while grey hairs make up less than 30 per cent of the head. Highlighting and lowlighting (see pp.98–99) are easy to apply and disguise the greying beautifully. Tinting the hair successfully becomes more difficult, however, as the white hairs start to make up the majority. As the hair becomes lighter, it helps if you use lighter and lighter colourants, as these blend more naturally with the skin and show a less obvious regrowth.

## GOING GREY

Individual hairs do not actually go grey – they turn white. The effect of grey is produced by the white hairs mixing with black or brown ones to give an overall appearance of grey. Blonde or red-haired women do not go grey at all in appearance – the hair simply seems to lighten at first.

The first white hairs can appear early on, but as you get into your 40s they normally start to grow apace. In some women grey hairs are evenly distributed throughout the head, although more usually they appear first at the temples and are most noticeable along the hairline. Some

Some women look stunning with natural greying or silvery-white hair; others look better with a tint. Experiment and see what suits you best. Rather than sticking to the style and colour that suited you in the past, look forward to a new way to appear beautiful in the future.

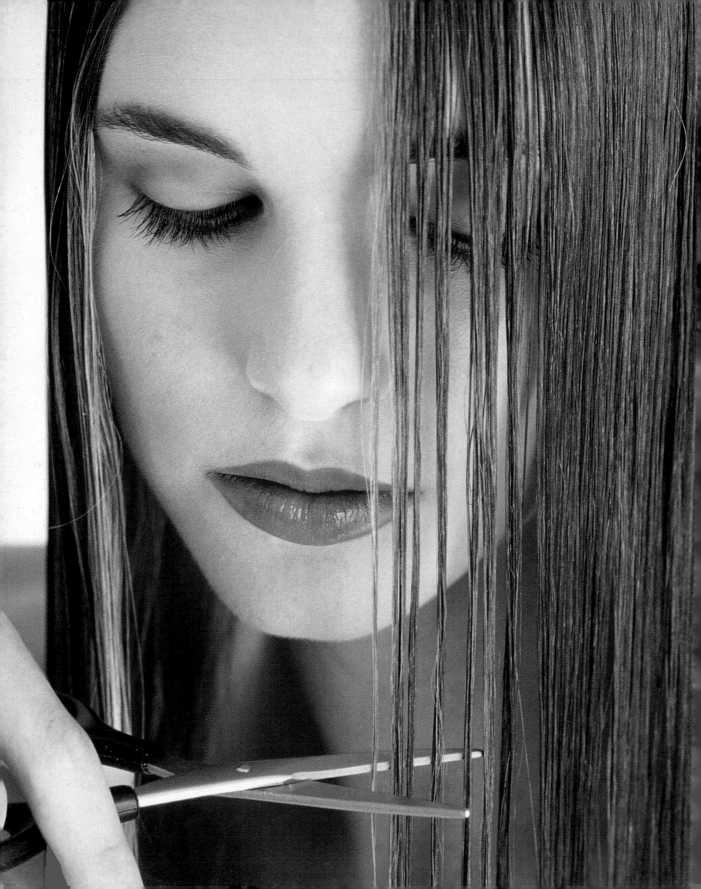

# HAIR
# Cuts

# Cutting YOUR HAIR

How you wear your hair says a great deal about your lifestyle and your personality. The hairstyle you choose is one of the strongest ways of making a statement about yourself.

Long hair is often considered to be the most feminine, and perhaps it is every woman's ideal to have a mass of flowing, wavy hair. But long hair needs a great deal of care: it was more suited to an era when women were decorative and did not go out to work. It takes longer to wash, shampoo and condition and much longer to dry.

While long hair that is well groomed and in good condition can look great, poorly cared-for long hair can look awful: the top part near the scalp may be pulled flat; the ends split and dry; and the hair can tangle and look unruly. The hair has been around for a considerable time, due to the sheer number of years it has taken to grow to that length, and it can become dry and porous at the ends, even when the roots are in good condition.

Mid-length hairstyles are often the most popular, because they give the illusion of length and can flow and wave, but may also be trimmed regularly. It is much easier to care for hair of this length.

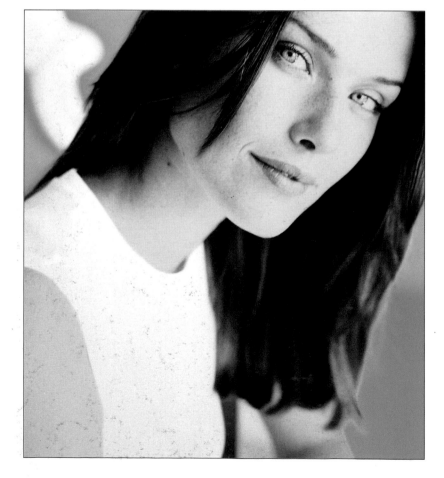

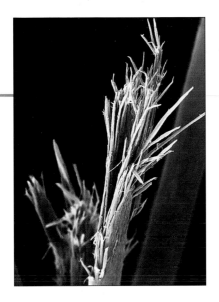

*Long hair tends to become dry and porous and will split at the ends. The only real cure for split ends is to have them cut off.*

Mid-length styles offer greater variety in terms of different cuts, and it is easy to change your hairstyle. When on the longer side, these styles still give you the opportunity to wear your hair in a variety of different ways.

Short styles can be dramatic and surprisingly feminine. If you have a good facial and skull structure, this may be the best choice for you, especially if you want to get rid of old, tinted or permed hair. When cutting hair very short, however, is is essential that you have a good stylist.

## HOW OFTEN TO CUT HAIR?

As a general rule, hair needs trimming every couple of months to remove split ends and tidy up the style.

The hair on your head grows at different rates in different places, so a haircut can get out of shape within a few weeks. For a very short stylish cut, the hair might need tidying up every four weeks. If you are trying to grow your hair long, then a trim every three months may be sufficient.

A good haircut, skilfully done, can transform a mediocre head of hair into something special. It's best to take care in finding someone to cut

your hair (see pp.108–109), as their skill will make all the difference. It is important to find a hairdresser who you like and feel relaxed with, and who will take time over your hair. It's no good going to the best cutter in London or New York if he is going to give you only 10 minutes, in an offhand manner, before rushing off to a fashion shoot.

**SAFETY TIP**
Never be tempted to cut your own hair or get a friend to cut it for you. Even cutting a fringe straight is a notoriously skilled job. In most cases you will need a good hairdresser to sort out the resulting disaster – it is better to make an appointment in the first place.

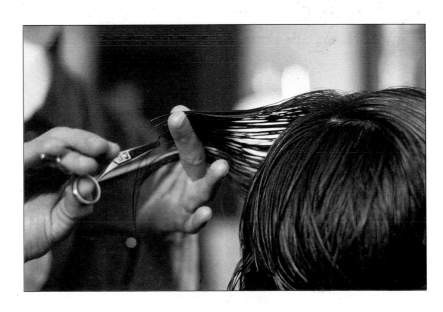

# Matching the shape
# OF YOUR FACE

**A** good hairdresser will look at the shape of your face before choosing a style for you. He or she will also look at the whole size and proportion of your body – if you have a small head and a tall, large-boned body, then a short, skull-hugging crop will look ridiculous.

**THE DIFFERENT FACE SHAPES**
You can establish your face shape by sitting in front of a mirror with your hair slicked back off your face. Draw the outline of your face on the mirror with a stick of old lipstick, following the contours exactly. Don't cheat! Then take a step back from the mirror and have a look. Your face should match one of these basic shapes:

- Square
- Round
- Oblong
- Heart
- Oval
- Pear
- Long

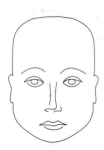

Square

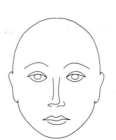

Round

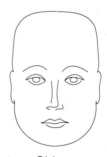

Oblong

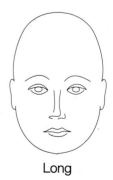

Long

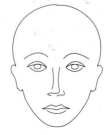

Heart

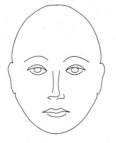

Oval

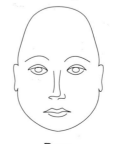

Pear

## SQUARE FACE

For a square face, choose a hairstyle with long layers, preferably one with soft waves and curls, to soften the outlines of the face. Part your hair on one side rather than in the centre and avoid a square-cut fringe.

## ROUND FACE

For a round face, a short haircut often looks good, especially one with a short fringe or hair swept back from the forehead, which tends to make the face look longer. Avoid very curly styles, or styles where the hair is pulled back from the face.

## OBLONG FACE

For an oblong face you need to give the illusion of width, so soften the effect with layers, or go for a bob with a fringe. Avoid styles without fringes and straight, long, one-length cuts.

## HEART FACE

For a heart-shaped face, cut a fringe or let the hair fall to conceal a widow's peak – or part the hair to make the most of it.

## OVAL FACE

An oval face is in many ways the perfect shape for any kind of hairstyle. If this is your face, experiment with the style of your choice – it should look great.

## PEAR-SHAPED FACE

For a pear-shaped face, try to create volume and bulk on top of the head to balance the lower part of the face.

## LONG FACE

For a long face, it is best to avoid long, straight hair. Use soft, feathered layers to create width at the side, and try a fringe to shorten the look of the face.

## IRREGULAR FEATURES

If your face is irregular in shape, choose soft styles and avoid harsh, geometric cuts.

## WEARING GLASSES

Always take spectacles to the salon with you to help blend your cut with them. Alternatively, choose new frames to suit a dramatic new hairstyle.

# Styling for specific problems:

| 1 | 2 | 3 | 4 | 5 | 6 |
|---|---|---|---|---|---|
| **PROMINENT NOSE** | **POINTED CHIN** | **LOW FOREHEAD** | **HIGH FOREHEAD** | **RECEDING CHIN** | **UNEVEN HAIRLINE OR WIDOW'S PEAK** |
| Choose a style that is soft and perhaps bulky at the back and sides, to draw attention away from the nose. | Style hair with width at the jawline to distract the eye. | Choose no fringe or a wispy fringe, not a thick fringe across the forehead. | This can be easily disguised with an appropriately cut fringe. | Choose a style that comes down below chin level, preferably with waves and curls. | Again, a fringe should conceal this problem. |

# Finding a good
# HAIRDRESSER

Try to choose a hairdresser who has been recommended by someone whose hair you like the look of. You might choose someone who has had experience of cutting hair in a major salon, but this does not necessarily mean that they will be better than someone from a small local salon. The most important thing is that you trust your hairdresser, that they make time to explain everything to you, and that they make you feel confident and valued.

### GETTING THE RIGHT CUT DEPENDS ON:

- The texture of your hair

- The shape of your face and head

- Your body shape and size

- Your lifestyle.

### BODY SHAPE AND LIFESTYLE FACTORS

If you are a new client, a good hairdresser should spend some time chatting to you and finding out what kind of person you are. He or she will want to see you when you come in and look at your hair in its natural state, before it has been shampooed.

Curly and straight hair will take different styles, and thick hair will cut differently from fine hair. They should also notice what clothes you are wearing and look at the proportions of your whole body standing up, not gowned in a chair, as your body style and shape will affect the volume and shape of your hair.

Wear the kind of clothes you normally wear – if you have to wear smart suits during the day, but like to look wild and go partying all evening, tell the hairdresser you want a hairstyle that's adaptable for many occasions. If you are a working mother with young children and never have time for yourself, you will probably ask for a style that is easy to maintain. If you need to look well groomed in your job, then you will require a different style from someone who wants to appear more natural.

### GOING FOR DRAMATIC CHANGE

A good hairdresser will not normally try to persuade you to do something dramatic straight away. They will often gain your confidence by doing your hair as you want it, or something close to your current style. Later, they may persuade you to try something more adventurous that they think will suit you or a new style that you have requested yourself.

New haircuts and styles can be a great shock. You yourself may love it, but hairdressers are quite used to women coming back to have their style changed because their boyfriend hates it. Everyone will comment on a new hairstyle and you need to have the confidence to carry off a dramatic change. If it is successful it can be a huge boost to the way you feel about yourself and to your morale, and a good hairdresser will appreciate this.

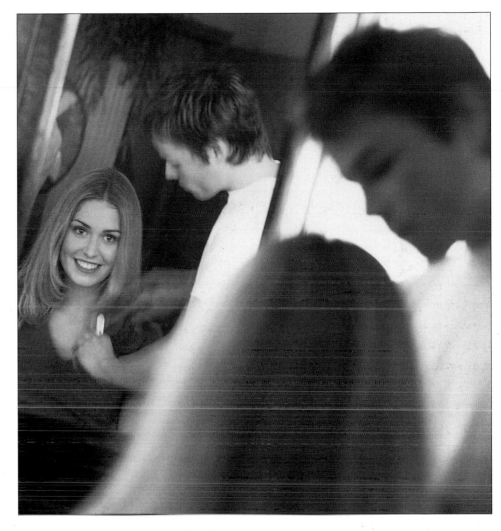

The secret of a good haircut is to make the best of your hair as it is. If your hair is naturally curly, it should be cut to emphasize the wave. If your hair is straight, it should be cut to hang straight. Problems arise when you want a hairstyle that doesn't suit your kind of hair. A good hairdresser will advise you of this and will usually recommend that the best way to feel happy with your hairstyle is to love your hair as it is, and not how you would like it to be.

Your hairdresser will probably ask you questions about whether you have ever coloured, tinted, permed or treated your hair and, if so, how long ago. Do try to be as honest as you can in your answers, as some treatments are not compatible with others and retreating hair that has previously been treated can cause damage. If you are having a tint or perm, your hairdresser should assess the porosity and elasticity of your hair and do a skin test first.

# Hair cutting techniques
## AND STYLES

The main hair cutting techniques are tapering, thinning and club cutting.

### TAPERING

This removes bulk from the hair and thins it, as well as removing length. It enables the hair to curl more readily and encourages any natural wave in the hair. Hair can be tapered either wet or dry. To taper dry hair the scissors are used in a slithering movement; with wet hair a razor is generally used, because scissors tend to tear the hair or lead to steps appearing in it when the wet hairs stick together.

### THINNING

Thinning removes natural bulk and weight from the hair and can help it to curl or lift, but does not alter the length. Scissors are used on dry hair, razors on wet. Hair should not be thinned at the hairline,

crown or along a parting, as the short ends of hair tend to stick up.

### CLUB CUTTING

This is a method of cutting the hair straight across, removing the length but retaining the bulk. It tends to discourage curling and is best used on straight hair. Club cutting is quite a skill, because while the hair is straight, the shape of the head is not, and the way that the hair hangs will affect its length.

### CUTTING FOR STYLE

Different cuts are used to create different styles of hair.

### BOB

Club cutting comes into its own to create the smooth, solid look of a bob. The hair is straight or curls under slightly and is club cut at the end to give it weight and bulk.

### LAYERED HAIR

Hair is thinned and tapered to create the layered look. Hair may be layered to make hair longer on the outside or on the inside, and may be cut to create many different effects.

### STYLES FOR LONG HAIR

Long hair is extremely versatile and can be worn in any number of different styles. Experiment with the ones described below and find out what suits your hair and the shape of your head and face.

### BRAID OR PLAIT

This can be perfectly simple or dressed up to look sophisticated. First, take a small section of hair on one side above your ear and separate it into two strands. Twist the strands together down to the nape of your neck, then pin and repeat

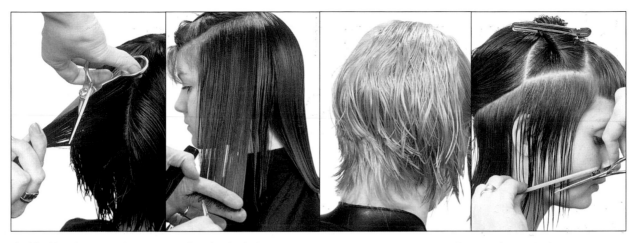

*A skilled hairdresser, using a variety of cutting techniques, will be able to create a number of different styles.*

on the other side. Now incorporate the twisted sections into a basic three-stranded plait: divide the hair into three equal strands, then bring the right strand over the centre one, the left over the centre, and then the right over the centre again. Continue to the end of the hair and secure with a covered band or clip bow.

### FRENCH BRAID

This sophisticated braid looks complex but gets easier with practice. Take a section of hair from the front of the head and divide it into three separate strands. Braid it once, taking the right over the centre, then the left over the centre, and then the right over the centre again.

Keeping hold of the braid with your fingers, use your thumbs to gather in additional hair from each side into the original strands. Continue braiding down the back of the head, incorporating more hair as you go. Secure with a covered band or clip.

### BUN

Smooth the hair into a ponytail, and place a bun-ring over it. Take about a third of the hair and wrap it round the bun-ring, then secure it with pins. Repeat with the other two-thirds of the hair.

To make a cameo braid around it, keep a long strand of hair separate from the ponytail from the outset. Then braid this in three strands and

wrap it around the outside of the bun.

### FRENCH PLEAT

Comb the hair on one side towards the back of the head. Smooth the hair across to the centre back and form the centre of the pleat by criss-crossing hair grips in a row from the crown downwards. Smooth the hair around from the other side, leaving the front end free, and tuck the ends under. Secure it with pins, then gently comb the front section up and around to merge with the top of the pleat. This style gives an elegant, sophisticated look, which can be worn every day, or dressed up for a special occasion.

# HAIRPIECES and accessories

If you want to create the illusion of long hair or wear a special hairstyle for a particular date, then a hairpiece may be the solution. Like hair extensions (see p.121), hairpieces can be made from real or synthetic hair. They come in every hair colour so that you can match the piece to your own hair. They have either a woven base (which may be machine- or hand-made) or a knotted base (which must be hand-knotted).

## USING A HAIRPIECE

To attach the hairpiece to the head, the hair must be brushed or combed in the direction of the style – into a ponytail, or up towards the top of the head. First, a square mesh of hair is sectioned off where the hairpiece is to go and is secured with hair grips. If the base of the hairpiece has a comb, then this can be pushed under the grips to hold it firmly; otherwise more hair grips are used to secure the hairpiece in position. The natural hair is then brushed or backcombed into place and the hair blended with that of the hairpiece, making sure that the base is camouflaged and that all hard lines and edges are blended in.

If you have never worn a hairpiece before, it is best to have it put in by a professional hairdresser. Once you have seen how it is done, you may easily be able to do this yourself at home, perhaps with the help of a friend.

A hairpiece can be set or blow-dried into the required style on a malleable block, if it is made of natural hair. If it is made of monofibre this cannot be done, but is unnecessary, as the style and curl are pre-set and will remain after washing.

## HAIR ACCESSORIES

Today there are many hair accessories that can help you make the most of your hair or brighten up your look for a special occasion. These include:

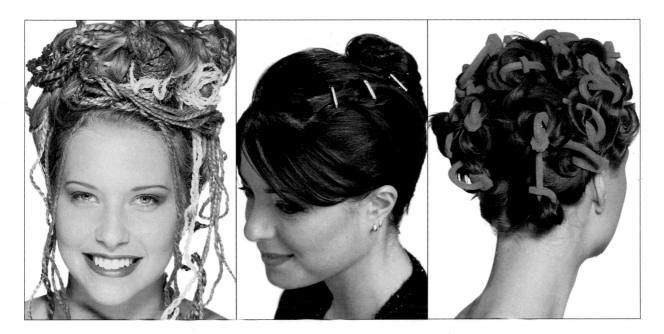

## SCRUNCHIES

These are elasticated bands covered with a tube of material, which ruches up when placed over a ponytail or braid. They come in a variety of fabrics, such as velvet, silk and soft chiffon, and can be embroidered with beads, sequins, and so on.

## BENDIES

Bendies are long pieces of flexible wire encased in fabric (often velvet or silk) that can be twisted into the hair in a variety of ways – as a band, braided into a ponytail or entwined around a bun. Some are plain while others are highly decorated.

## BOWS

These can be tailored or floppy and are often made from materials like silk and velvet. They can also be attached to a slide.

## HEADBANDS

From a simple Alice band to something much more dramatic and daring, headbands can be used to hold the hair back from the face. They come in a variety of widths and fabrics.

## SLIDES, COMBS AND PINS

These are used to hold hair in place when wearing it up, and can also be used instead of bands or scrunchies to secure a ponytail, plaits or braids. Jewelled hair clips or slides with bows or artificial flowers are great for dressing up the hair for parties or special occasions.

Combs of many different kinds can be used to secure the hair. Some combs swivel and lock into place, while others simply slide into the hair to secure decorative items such as flowers or jewellery.

## SNOODS

These may be old-fashioned, but they can still look great secured around braids, buns and chignons.

# PERMING

Perming is most often used to wave or curl the hair. The resulting style is permanent because the structure of the hair is altered, and the wave or curl can only be removed again if it is left to grow out or the hair is re-permed.

## HAIR CHEMISTRY

It helps to know a little about hair chemistry to understand how perms work. Hair is formed of keratin, a protein made up of amino acids containing carbon, hydrogen, oxygen, nitrogen

and sulphur. The amino acids are joined up end-to-end to form long chains called polypeptides, and these have a large number of cross-linkages between the different chains. The main bonds are formed by two sulphur atoms linking together two adjacent polypeptide chains. These linkages are like the rungs of a ladder

and can only be broken by chemical treatment.

Most hair contains about 4–5 per cent sulphur, although natural red hair may have up to 8 per cent, making it more resistant and difficult to treat. It also contains salt or electrostatic bonds between the polypeptide chains, which are easily broken by weak acids and alkalis. Finally, there are hydrogen bonds between the coils of a polypeptide chain and between different chains. These bonds, while weak,

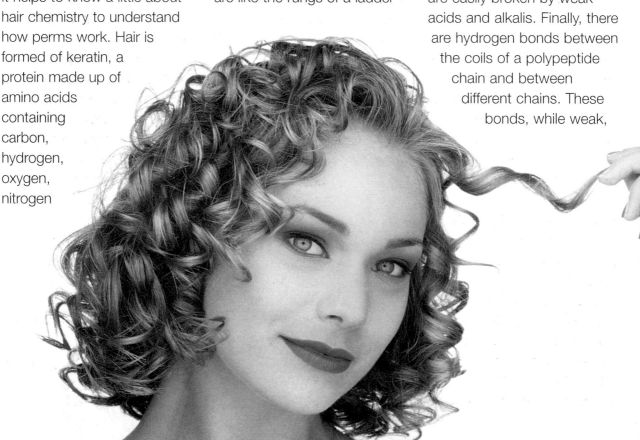

are very plentiful. Hydrogen bonds can be broken by water and most weak chemicals. They come into play when the hair is 'set' in rollers and when heat is used in blow-drying and heated rollers, and they help to give bounce and body to hair.

## PERMING STAGES

There are three stages in perming, known as softening, moulding and neutralizing.

## SOFTENING

In softening, the perm lotion is applied to the hair. It contains a substance called ammonium thioglycolate, which is highly alkaline with a pH of about 9–9.5. This attacks and breaks the strong cross-linkages in the hair, which are known as sulphur bonds. Usually about 60–70 per cent of these are broken.

Acid perms contain another chemical, glycerol thioglycolate, which has a pH value of about 4. However, an alkali has to be mixed with this before application of the lotion, to lift the hair cuticle and allow the perm lotion to penetrate the cortex. Although these perms are called 'acid', they are not actually acid on application, but simply less alkaline than the ammonium thioglycolate perms. In acid perms only about 10 per cent of the sulphur bonds are broken. While acid perms are more gentle on the hair, there is a fairly high rate of allergic reaction to them: about 20 per cent of applications produce contact dermatitis.

The chemical process involved in breaking the sulphur bonds is called reduction. During this process the thioglycolate adds hydrogen atoms which attach themselves to the sulphur atoms that normally bond to one another, forming the cross-chain bonds and breaking them down. If the perm lotion is left on too long, permanent damage results.

## MOULDING

During the second stage the softened hair is moulded as it is wrapped round rollers. The tension should be such that the hair stretches slightly, allowing the polypeptide chains of the hair protein to slide past one another. Care has to be taken not to wind the curler too tightly, as this will stretch the hair – especially when it is wet – and then damage will be done. The size and shape of the rollers dictates the tightness of the curl.

## NEUTRALIZING

After moulding, the perm lotion is rinsed off the hair. The final stage is neutralizing the perm. The polypeptide chains have to be locked into their new positions by removing the hydrogen atoms, which stop the sulphur bonds from forming. This is done by adding an oxidizing agent, such as hydrogen peroxide (usually in a strength of about 6 per cent) or sodium perborate (generally 5 per cent). The oxygen bonds with the hydrogen to make water, and the sulphur bonds re-form, locking the hair in the new position.

As with permanent hair tinting or colouring, the hair should always be tested for porosity before perming. Hair that has been damaged by bleaching, colouring or previous perming may not be strong enough to sustain another perm.

# TYPES of perm

The size and shape of the rollers or rods used for perming, and the way in which the hair is wound around them, will affect the end result. The smaller the rods or rollers used, the tighter the perm will be.

## BODY PERM

In a body perm, large rollers are used to create a soft, wave-like effect and to add volume and bounce, rather than curls, to the hair.

## ROOT PERM

This adds lift and volume to the root area only. It gives height and fullness, and is therefore ideal for short hair that tends to go flat.

## PIN-CURL PERM

This gives soft, natural waves and curls, by pinning curls on the head instead of using rollers in the hair.

## STACK PERM

A stack perm gives wave and volume to hair that has been cut to one length, by means of different-sized curlers. The hair on top of the head is usually left unpermed, while the middle and ends are given curl and movement.

## SPIRAL PERM

This creates spiralling curls or ringlets and is made by using vertical rather than horizontal rods. The mass of curls gives volume and makes the hair look thicker. This method is also used for perming long hair, as the normal winding of locks many times around a curler would produce a tighter curl at the hair tips and a very loose curl at the root end. Also, lotions do not penetrate through a thickly wound curler, so the process does not provide a satisfactory result for long hair.

## SPOT PERM

A spot perm is applied to one particular area, such as the fringe or the side areas around the face, in order to give lift.

## WEAVE PERM

This is the term used when some sections of hair are

**DID YOU KNOW ?**
Modern perms were invented by A.F. Willett who devised the 'cold permanent wave' treatment in 1934. Since then, the formula has been improved and new, sophisticated techniques have made the perm a versatile styling option.

permed and others are not, giving a combination of texture and natural-looking body and bounce.

## THE PROBLEM OF REGROWTH

Obviously the new hair that grows through after a perm will have the old, straight texture. This is not usually noticeable at first, but if you have had a tight perm it will become obvious after about six weeks to two months. The areas of new growth can be re-permed if a barrier is created over the permed hair, either by using a thick barrier cream or a plastic protector. This is usually skilled work and should only be attempted in a salon.

# HOME perms

**HOME PERMS**

It is possible to perm your hair at home, but it is much easier and more reliable to have it done in a salon. The chemicals used can be dangerous, especially if left on the scalp for too long or if they get into your eyes, and it is difficult to wind the hair evenly on the rollers without help. Speed and skill are essential, too. In the salon there may be two people carrying out the task, who will have a good view of your whole head and will not have problems reaching difficult areas. At home you may be struggling with a mirror and clumsy fingers, and be unable to see exactly what you're doing. If you do use a home perm, try to get a friend to help you, and carefully follow the instructions printed on the packet. You must also have a reliable timer, and remember to remove the pins and curlers in the same order that you put them in.

There is also a greater choice of types of curl and degrees of perm with a professional perm, and it is easier for the hairdresser to do the essential tests. An experienced hairdresser will not try to perm hair that obviously will not take it, but many mistakes can be made at home. When done badly, or put on hair that is already porous or damaged, a perm can be dangerous: it can harm the hair, making it lank and lifeless, or even make the hairs break off near the scalp. Burns to the scalp from the chemicals used can even cause permanent hair loss in some cases.

If you are in any doubt at all about how your hair will react to a perm, always consult a professional hairdresser for their opinion and follow their advice. This is especially important if you have never permed your hair before or it has been permed recently.

## Tips on home perming:

| 1 | 2 | 3 | 4 | 5 | 6 |
|---|---|---|---|---|---|
| Read all the instructions on the packaging first and follow them to the letter. | Remember to do a test curl to check whether your hair is suitable. | Make sure that you have enough rollers and pins, and have everything you need to hand. | Try to enlist the help of a friend who can stop you panicking, pass you items that you need and wind the rollers on those parts of the head you can't reach. | Timing is of the essence, so don't be tempted to unwind the rollers too soon or to leave them on longer than directed in the instructions. | Never perm your hair if there are any sores, cuts or abrasions on the scalp. |

# HAVING a perm

## THE PERMING PROCESS

1   Sometimes the hair is cut before, sometimes after, a perm. Thinned or tapered hair is easier to wind round the rods or rollers.

2   The hair is shampooed, rinsed and then dabbed partially dry with a towel. Conditioner should not be used, as this will coat the hair and help prevent penetration of the hair shaft.

3   Barrier cream is usually applied to the hairline to protect the skin in case any of the perm lotion drips down on to it.

4   The hair is normally divided into sections – sometimes as many as nine – to make it easier to wind the hair on to the rods or rollers. If your hair is particularly short, thick or abundant, the hairdresser may need to divide the hair into even more sections to produce the desired result.

5   Cotton wool is fixed around the hair line. The hair is usually wound first, while still damp from shampooing, and the lotion is then applied. The hair is then wound evenly around the rod or roller and pinned or otherwise secured into place. The tension should not be too great or this can pull out individual hairs and cause 'pull burns' on the scalp.

6   When the lotion has been applied, a second application is generally applied immediately afterwards. The rods are checked at regular intervals – normally every three to five minutes.

7   When the perm has developed, the hair is rinsed thoroughly in warm water. Care should be taken to prevent any water running into the eyes.

8   Excess water is removed from the hair. Cotton wool is then put around the hairline to protect the skin.

9   The neutralizer is applied as a cream, foam or liquid. It may be used straight from the container or applied with a brush or sponge. It is then left for the recommended time (usually five minutes).

10   The rods should be removed carefully without dragging the hair.

11   A further application of neutralizer is dabbed over the hair, then left for another five minutes or so. The hair should then be rinsed thoroughly.

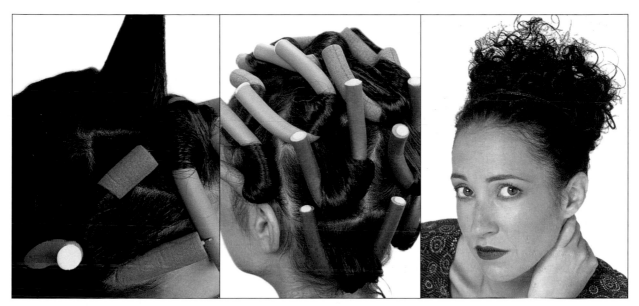

*A perm can transform your hair into a mass of glorious curls.*

After a perm it takes about 48 hours for the keratin in the hair to harden again. During this time the hair is vulnerable to damage and must be treated with care. Resist shampooing, brushing, vigorous combing, blow-drying or setting it, as these may cause the perm to drop. After a while, the perm will tend to soften, especially if the hair is long. Hair will be drier and more porous and will need more conditioning than untreated hair.

Care must be taken in drying the hair immediately after a perm, as the perm will not fully take effect until the hair has dried. Vigorous blow-drying or towelling will tend to undo some of the curl, so treat the hair gently.

# Post-perm tips:

| 1 | 2 | 3 | 4 | 5 |
|---|---|---|---|---|
| Don't wash newly permed hair for 48 hours afterwards, as this can cause some of the perm to drop out. | Use shampoos and conditioners specially designed for permed hair. | When combing, always use a wide-toothed comb and work from the ends upwards. Never brush the hair. | Blot wet hair dry before styling it to prevent the hair from stretching. | Avoid using too much heat on permed hair – if possible, allow it to dry naturally after shampooing and conditioning. |

# STRAIGHTENING and relaxing

Straightening or relaxing hair is the most drastic of all the processes used on hair and great care must be taken not to leave it irreparably damaged. The technique is often used on African Caribbean hair and is suitable for very tight curls or frizzy hair. If you want to straighten Caucasian curls, it is better to have a 'reverse perm', in which the hair is held straight after using normal perm lotions.

Calcium hydroxide, potassium hydroxide and sodium

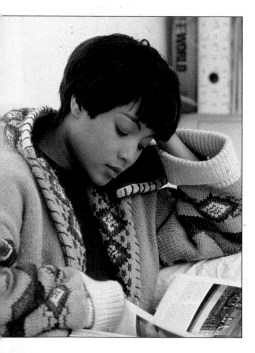

hydroxide are all strong alkalis used to straighten hair. They have a pH of 10–14. Sodium hydroxide (usually known as caustic soda or lye) is the most commonly used substance and is only allowed to be used in a concentration of 4.5 per cent in the UK, while in the US the permitted level is as high as 10 per cent. Relaxers also often contain moisturizers, conditioning agents and skin coolers to help lessen skin irritation.

The process is different from perming and involves more complex chemical reactions. The sulphide bonds are broken down and one of the sulphur atoms is removed, producing a new amino acid called lanthionine. The hair then rebonds with a single sulphur bond. The process does not require a neutralizer, as the reaction stops when the sodium hydroxide is rinsed from the hair and an acid shampoo is applied. When the hair has dried, it should remain in its new, straightened shape. Once

hair has been chemically relaxed, it cannot be permed, as it has a new structure and cannot re-form the normal disulphide bonds.

Relaxing should only ever be done by a skilled hairdresser who has experience of using this technique. As a general rule, relaxers are manufactured in three strengths: super – for strong, resistant or coarse hair; regular – for normal hair; and mild – for fine or colour-treated hair. The strong varieties can have twice the concentration of the mild. Use of too strong a product can lead to serious hair and scalp damage.

As with perms, there will be a problem of regrowth and the new hair may need to be retreated. Even more so than with a perm, it is vital to protect the hair that has already been relaxed. Great care should be taken in conditioning it, as it will have become more porous and will tend to dry out and become brittle.

# HAIR extensions

It is easy to decide to change your hair from long to short – you simply go and have a great haircut. But what if you want to change your image by going from short to long? There is a way round having to grow your hair long over a number of years: you can try hair extensions. These can be made of real hair or, more commonly, of synthetic fibre which is very hard to distinguish from the real thing. Fixing these extensions is a highly skilled and time-consuming job, but it can produce great results.

## THE WEAVING PROCESS

Small meshes of the natural hair are sectioned off and the long strands of the hair extension are woven into them, and are then fixed with a glue. With real hair extensions, the weaving has to be very secure. Artificial fibre extensions are sealed into the hair with heat which melts and fuses the fibre, thus enabling it to be more firmly anchored. Whichever type of extension is used, its maximum life is approximately five months. This is because the natural hair is growing at roughly 1cm ($\frac{1}{2}$in) per month, and as it grows the join becomes visible and looks unsightly. It is, however, possible for a hairdresser to refit hair extensions after that period of time.

You should never go for hair extensions that are more than twice the length of your natural hair, as their weight could damage your own hair. Obviously, harsh brushing or tugging on the hair should be avoided, as it may weaken the bonds that hold the extension to your natural hair. Be sure that the salon gives you information on after-care, as this is extremely important if you wish hair extensions to last. You should also not have extensions fitted if your hair is in poor condition or chemically damaged, as this will break the hair further. Natural hair extensions can be set, curled, bleached and highlighted, like real hair.

## Tips for managing hair extensions:

| 1 | 2 | 3 | 4 | 5 | 6 |
|---|---|---|---|---|---|
| Don't go for high ponytails, buns or Heidi-style plaits, because these will tend to show the natural hair underneath, which may look different from the hair. | When brushing, use a soft bristle brush rather than brushes with plastic or metal teeth. | Gently tie your hair back when sleeping to avoid tangling your hair and the extensions. | Never comb your natural hair from the root ends as you will damage the joints. | Chlorine will not affect your hair extension if you love to swim, but protect it from the heat of a sauna by pinning it up and wrapping it in a towel. | If you care for your hair extension well, it will look great for months. |

# Questions

## AND ANSWERS

**Q** I am suspicious of all the claims made for expensive shampoos and conditioners, so I just use standard cheap shampoo from the local chemist as I tend to shampoo my hair several times a week. Recently, though, I have noticed that my hair seems to have become dry and frizzy. Should I change my shampoo or should I use a conditioner?

**A** If you are buying cheap shampoo, it may be that you are using one with a detergent that is too strong, especially if you wash your hair frequently. This tends to remove too much sebum from the hair and make it dry and porous. Look for a shampoo that contains sodium or ammonium laureth sulphate, rather than only the stronger lauryl sulphate. Using conditioner should definitely help, by restoring lost oil to the hair. Look for one for dry or damaged hair and, if the condition is really bad, consider trying a one-off deep-conditioning treatment, such as henna wax.

**Q** My hair is really greasy and, no matter how often I wash it, it looks lank and dreadful the next day. I read somewhere that frequent washing makes hair look worse, as it stimulates the scalp to produce even more oil. I tried leaving it, but after three days I couldn't bear it, so I washed it again. What should I do? I am 19 by the way.

**A** If you use a mild 'frequent-wash' shampoo, then daily washing should not harm your hair. Massage the scalp only very gently when washing, and keep the water fairly cool. Many young people do tend to produce a lot of sebum, but this usually settles down with time. It's a myth that a fat-rich diet tends to make you produce more sebum, so you don't have to cut out all chocolate and fat, but it wouldn't harm you to eat more oils, fruit, vegetables and lean meats. You could also try a different hairstyle – long hair tends to get pulled flat at the roots, while short hair often has more lift and curl, which may disguise the problem.

**Q** I'm fed up with my dead-straight hair and am thinking of having a perm, but I'm hesitating because I'm afraid it will damage my hair.

**A** If you have a perm done professionally, it should not cause serious damage to your hair, although it will usually become drier and you will have to take more time conditioning and looking after it. This depends, however, on how curly you want it to be and whether you will want to go on having your hair permed regularly. The best thing to do is to talk to your hairdresser and then, if you feel convinced, take the plunge! You can always grow it out again eventually.

**Q** I've seen people wearing sleek, wet-looking hair – how do they achieve that sort of look?

**A** Wet-look hair relies on modern styling products to create the right finish. Serums and gels are ideal for achieving a glossy, slick finish, while waxes and pomades used over several or more strands can define the texture and give a hint of wetness. The hair should usually be allowed to dry naturally to make the most of the curl; or, if your hair is straight, comb the product through to give that just-out-of–the-shower look.

**Q** My hair tends to fly all over the place and my hairdresser suggested hair spray, but I don't want my hair to look set rigid, like a helmet. He said that the modern hair sprays don't give this effect. Is he right?

**A** Many modern hair sprays use new, more flexible polymers that do not give as strong a hold as the standard products. These may be more suitable if you want a natural look. The secret is to keep the spray container a reasonable distance from your head and let the drops fall gently on to it. Use hair spray sparingly at first, then use a bit more when you gain confidence, until you find the right amount to achieve the look you want. You might also like to try the anti-static conditioners that are now available.

**Q** I am breastfeeding my baby and have noticed that my hair, which used to be curly, has gone straight and a lot of it seems to be falling out. Is this normal?

**A** Probably what you are seeing is the normal hair loss that may occur after the baby's birth when extra hair is lost. Some women do notice a change in the curliness of their hair while breastfeeding, possibly due to high oestrogen levels (this also sometimes happens during the teenage years when hormone levels change). However, it should go back to normal eventually. Do take care to eat enough iron-rich foods, proteins and vitamins, and check that you are not anaemic after the birth.

**Q** I have noticed my first grey hairs, and as there aren't many of them I am currently pulling them out. A friend said that I shouldn't do this, as the hairs won't grow back properly. Is that correct?

**A** Pulling out hair with tweezers may damage or distort the hair follicle, and on rare occasions it may even become infected. However, initially plucking hairs will stimulate new growth for a short while. But it's not a good idea to pull out white hairs, especially on a regular basis, as they will simply be replaced by more. If you really hate the white hairs, try using a temporary hair colour. Alternatively, you could try having your hair highlighted, which would disguise the white hairs, especially as you get more of them.

**Q** I have been told that I have alopecia. I don't have any bald patches, so can this be correct?

**A** Yes, is the short answer. The condition to which you refer, with bald patches, is alopecia areata. It is commonly abbreviated, incorrectly, simply to alopecia, although medically this term refers to all forms of hair loss. So you may be suffering from a very mild condition, such as a little extra hair loss following a high temperature, but this is still called alopecia. Rarely, alopecia areata can sometimes lead to thinning rather than patchy loss of hair.

**Q** Why do most men go bald while most women don't?

**A** Male-pattern baldness is a genetically inherited condition. It is the male hormone testosterone that causes the problem. A man inherits the ability to transform this hormone into another form of itself, called dihydrotestosterone or DHT. When this happens, the DHT settles in the hair follicles on the top of the head, where the hairs are able to accept this hormone, and then the hair starts to degenerate. The process is normally slow and takes several years. Women, however, are more protected from balding because their oestrogen levels are higher, which helps to neutralize the effects of testosterone.

**Q** I live in a big city, but I've been told that if I want to see a trichologist I will have to travel 65 km (40 miles) to find one. Why are there so few about?

**A** Trichology is a very specialized subject, and for this reason there are not a large number of trichologists in clinical practice. The Institute of Trichologists (London), founded in 1902, is well established, but nevertheless remains small. Not all trichologists go into clinical practice, however. Some work in education; others act as advisers to industry, hospitals or universities; some work in manufacturing; and others work in the law courts, giving expert advice on all sorts of cases involving the hair or scalp (from hairdressing problems and accidents to actual bodily harm and even murder). For this reason, there may be areas of a country where those in clinical practice are a bit thin on the ground. Contact the Institute of Trichologists or the International Association of Trichologists, who can advise you on your nearest practising member.

# Index

## A

Acid perms 115
Adolescence 18
Afro Caribbean hair 20, 25, 81
  Colouring 100
Ageing 18, 54, 55–56, 101
Alcohol 50
Alkali (see bleach)
Alopecia 58–64
  Androgenic 58–59
  Areata 60–61, 62
  Traction 20, 61

## B

Babies 16
Backcombing 40
Baldness (see hair loss,
  alopecia)
Bleach 30, 74, 91
Blowdrying 38–39
Bob 110
Braid 110
Brushes 40
Brushing 40–41
Bun 110

## C

Cancer 66
Chlorine 30
Clips, hair 45
Club cutting 110
Colour (natural) 80–81
Colourings 83–89
  Permanent 90–91
  Quasi-permanent 90
  Semi-permanent 89

Temporary 88–89
Conditioners 34–35
Contraceptive pills (see oral
  contraceptives)
Combs 41
  Afro 25
Cornrows 45
Cortex 14
Corticosteroids (see
  steroids)
Cowlick 17
Crown 16, 17
Cuticle 14, 16, 20
Cutting 46, 104–107

## D

Dandruff 72–73
  Anti-dandruff agents 30
Depilation 75
Depilatory creams 75
Dermatitis 69
  Seborrhoeic 72
Diet 50–53
Dressing creams 42
Dry hair 24
Drying 38–39

## E

Eczema 68–69, 72
Effleurage 36
Electrolysis 71

## F

Finger drying 39
Follicle 14, 15
Friction (massage) 36

## G

Gel, hair 44
GLA, gamma linoleic acid 64
Greasy hair 24
Green tea 64
Grey (white) hair 18, 55, 101

## H

Hair
  Colour 80–83
  Excessive 74
  Extensions 121
  Growth cycle 18–19
  Pubic 18
  Root 14
  Shaft 14
  Structure 14–15
  Transplants 63
  Unwanted 74
Hair loss 18, 58–63, 66
  Treatments 62–63
Hairdressers 108
Hairdriers 38–39
Hairpiece 112
Hairspray 42–43
Headbands 45, 113
Headlice (see lice)
Henna 86, 94–95
Herbs 29
Highlighting 98–99
Hormonal changes 18, 55
Hormone disorders 59, 74
Hormone replacement therapy
  (HRT) 55, 59
Hydrogen peroxide 74, 90–91

**I**

Impetigo 70
Infections, scalp 70
Iron 50, 52

**K**

Keratin 14
Ketaconazole 64, 70

**L**

Lanolin 20
Lanugo hair 16
Layering 111
Lice (head) 70–71
Lowlighting 98–99

**M**

Male pattern baldness
  (androgenic alopecia) 54, 58–59
Massage (head) 36
Medulla 14
Melanin 82
Menopause 19, 59
Minoxydil 61, 62
Mousse 42

**N**

Neutralisation (of perms) 115
Nits 70–71

**O**

Oily hair (see greasy hair)
Oral contraceptives 59
Oriental hair 20, 81

**P**

Perms 114–119
  Home 117
Petrissage 36
PH balance (in shampoos) 3
Pheomelanin 82
Pill, the (see oral contraceptives)

Pins 45, 113
Plaiting 110
Plucking 76
Pollution 54
Porosity (of hair) 92
Pregnancy 18
  And hair loss 18
Products (hair) 42–43
Proteins:
  In diet 50
  In shampoos 28
Psoriasis 68
PUVA 63

**R**

Redhead 81
Relaxing hair 120
Restructurants 35
Retouching 91
Reverse perms 120
Ringworm 70
Rollers 45

**S**

Salons 108
Scalp, disorders of 68–69
Sebaceous cyst 69
Sebaceous gland 16
Seborrhoeic eczema (see
  eczema, seborrhoeic)
Sebum 16
Setting 44–45
Shampoos 26–27
  Additives in 28–31
Shaving 75
Shine enhancers 42
Skin test 93
Soap 32
Split ends 104–105
Steroids 61, 62
Straightening 120
Strand test 92

Stress 54
Styling 44–45
Sunscreens 46–47

**T**

Tapering 110
Terminal hair 17
Texture (of hair) 18
Tinting (see colouring)
Thinning 110
Tongs 45
Trichologists 56–57

**U**

Ultraviolet rays (UVBs) 46–47, 63

**V**

Vegetable dyes 96–97
Vegetarians 50–51
Vellus hair 17
Vitamins 52–53
  A 52
  B6 64
  B12 52
  C 50

**W**

Waxes, hair 42
Waxing 76
Whorl 17
Widow's peak 17
Wigs 67

**Z**

Zinc 50, 52, 63
Zinc pyrithione 30

**With thanks to Peter Legg of Holistic Hair and Beauty at 186–188 West End Lane, West Hampstead, London, NW6 1SG, 020 7435 7514**

## Bibliography

*Hairstyles*, Jacki Wadeson, Lorenz Books, 1994

*The Art of Hair Colouring*, David Adams and Jacki Wadeson, Macmillan, 1998

*Professional Hairdressing*, Martin Green, Lesley Howson, Leo Palladino and the Hairdressing Training Board, Macmillan 1994

*Afro Hair – A Salon Handbook*, Phillip Hatton, Blackwell Scientific Publications, 1994

*Perming and Straightening*, Phillip Hatton and Lesley Hatton, Blackwell Scientific Publications, 1993

*Hairdressing, the Complete Guide*, Peter Cutting and Renie Ross, Addison Wesley Longman Limited 1996